HEALTHY VESSELS

A Christian Guide for a Healthy Lifestyle

Jim Williamson, BS, MA, EdS

iUniverse, Inc.
Bloomington

Healthy Vessels
A Christian Guide for a Healthy Lifestyle

iUniverse books may be ordered through booksellers or by contacting:

iUniverse
1663 Liberty Drive
Bloomington, IN 47403
www.iuniverse.com
1-800-Authors (1-800-288-4677)

ISBN: 978-1-4502-8471-4 (pbk)
ISBN: 978-1-4502-8475-2 (cloth)
ISBN: 978-1-4502-8472-1 (ebk)

Printed in the United States of America

iUniverse rev. date: 3/28/11

I can do all things through Christ which strengtheneth me.
—Philippians 4:13

Acknowledgments

A special thank-you goes to the following individuals and classes who have inspired and supported me in the writing of this book.

My wife, Terri, has spent endless hours editing and proofreading my writing. Her input on relevant ideas was immeasurable. She helped as an assistant in the Healthy Vessels classes, helped tabulate results, performed clerical tasks and provided support to ensure that class operations ran smoothly. Without her help, the Healthy Vessels project would have been impossible.

My daughter, Julie Williamson-Wright, was instrumental in providing the technological expertise necessary to utilize available resources for classroom instruction and presentations. Her willingness to invest countless hours in formatting and preparing this document for publication was critical in meeting key deadlines.

The members of Cornerstone Baptist Church who participated in the first three Healthy Vessels classes during 2009 and the class members at Tri-City Baptist Church in Port Charlotte, Florida, were instrumental in demonstrating the positive results that can occur when health habits are changed. Participants lost over a thousand pounds, eliminated prescribed medications, and experienced a wide variety of positive health benefits. These positive benefits served as evidence that others could benefit from this program in the future.

I dedicate this book to my wife, Terri; my daughters, Jo Lynn and Julie; and my granddaughters, Megan, Madison, and Mackenzie.

CONTENTS

PART I:

GAINING PERSPECTIVE

Preface

Nearly eight years ago, I began to experience some deteriorating health conditions that I first diagnosed as "growing older." I was upset that my blood pressure was higher and that a physician had recommended that I begin taking blood pressure medication. I had never had high blood pressure before, and I was bewildered about my present situation. I was also having continual pain in my left thumb. After I had X-rays taken, I was told that I had arthritis. When I received this news, my perception was that arthritis was a symptom of old age. Besides the high blood pressure and arthritis, I just did not feel healthy. Due to past knee injuries and surgeries, I had always been concerned that someday I would be a candidate for a knee replacement. Occasionally my knee would just "go out," and this intensified my fears of a knee surgery, which I really dreaded thinking about. Like many people, I had frequent colds and experienced recurring allergy symptoms. My weight was higher than I believed it should be. I occasionally took antacid pills, and I would periodically experience a sore neck. My back would often be out of alignment, causing me pain. Things were not going well!

When I began reflecting on all of these undesirable symptoms, I did not want to accept that these physical symptoms were the result of getting older. I wanted to believe that my lifestyle was the problem because that was the only thing that I could possibly change. At minimum, I knew that my weight gain was connected to how I was eating. I thought that just maybe some of the other symptoms I was experiencing were connected to lifestyle choices. My only hope was that I might experience better health if I changed my present habits because I knew that I could not change my age! Since I sincerely wanted to experience a new level of health, I had only one real option to impact my present health: taking a hard look at my lifestyle. I thought if I was willing to make some lifestyle changes, it just might impact my overall health.

Once I made the decision to pursue a plan of healthy eating and exercise, it was my intent to discover if my lifestyle changes could alleviate some of the symptoms that I was experiencing. And when I began researching positive health choices, I realized I was not making these healthy choices for myself. At the beginning, my focus was on losing weight, reducing my blood pressure, and strengthening my right knee in order to delay or eliminate the need for a knee replacement.

During the next twelve weeks, I was able to experience positive changes beyond my expectations. The high blood pressure disappeared; the acid reflux stopped; my right knee stopped "going out" on me; my allergies disappeared; and the arthritis symptoms in my left hand disappeared along with my lower back problems. I have been able to avoid any kind of illness for more than eight years. It would be difficult to convince me that these results have been a coincidence. I developed the Healthy Vessels program for the purpose of forwarding information to others so that they may also be able to regain their health.

This book was written in response to the obesity crisis in America, which threatens to financially bankrupt our national health care system. In addition to the financial peril, this crisis is responsible for much physical suffering and thousands of debilitating diseases and premature deaths.

It is of particular concern to me that so many Christians are active participants in the unhealthy life choices that contribute to this present crisis. Even though it is sometimes difficult to do, I believe that Christians have a responsibility to live by example. The Bible tells us clearly that we are not to follow the ways of the world, that we must take care of our bodies, and that we are to glorify God in our body and in our spirit. This is unfortunately not the standard being followed by many Christians. When we allow ourselves to eat and drink in a manner that promotes disease and related health problems, as I did, the standard that is exemplified in the Bible is compromised. In the area of health and lifestyle choices, statistics reveal that Christians practice the same unhealthy habits that the world does, and Christians are also experiencing the negative consequences of their unhealthy choices.

It concerns me that many Christians are more than eager to discuss certain habits that abuse our bodies without addressing diet and exercise deficiencies. Issues such as the evils of alcohol, tobacco, and drugs are discussed freely in many Christian churches; however, the abuse of food—and the resulting health problems—are often not discussed at all. *I believe that abuse is abuse, regardless of the source.* The irony is that most of the prayer requests each week in church are health-related. For a three-month period of time, I recorded data regarding the prayer requests that were made each week in our church. I documented that each week between 80 and 90 percent of all prayer requests in our church were health-related. I still document the prayer requests periodically, and this statistic still holds true.

Yet solutions and practices intended to avoid or reduce one's risk of developing certain health problems are almost never discussed. This silence occurs at the same time that some health professional believe up to 85 percent of all debilitating diseases are caused by lifestyle choices. Millions of Americans are living unhealthy lifestyles, and many of these people are Christians. Since at least two-thirds of all Americans are practicing habits detrimental to their health, it seems that this is a relevant subject area to address. It is like the elephant in the room!

This book is intended to provide some direction for both the secular world and Christians. My hope is that in the midst of our present health crisis in America, Christians will assume greater responsibility for their health and choose to set a better example. Adopting more self-control and discipline with respect to our health is consistent with Christian principles. These two qualities are always discussed positively in the Bible. The reality that more than two-thirds of all adults in this country are either overweight or obese is evidence that both self-control and discipline have been compromised by many people. Being overweight is a significant risk factor for developing debilitating diseases. Getting control of this visible and measurable health risk factor is a good starting point to begin the journey of establishing higher health standards. My experience is that this can be done. The Healthy Vessels program can show you how to make positive lifestyle changes!

Introduction

Except for an emergency surgery at birth because I was unable to digest food properly, I experienced pretty good health throughout most of my young life. In high school, I was the school record holder in the mile run and was the district champion in the half-mile run. I also made claim to the unofficial national high school record in the fifty-mile run. I lettered in cross country during college and placed in an AAU marathon race (26.2 miles).

However, like many adults, I failed to keep a firm grip on my health. In my early twenties, I participated in adult athletic teams and tore the anterior cruciate ligament (ACL) in my right knee during a basketball game. Two knee operations would follow during the next decade. I developed poor eating and drinking habits like those that are so prevalent in our culture. My body weight ballooned to an unhealthy 232 pounds. Though in high school I had been a six-foot-three-inch distance runner weighing in at 147 pounds, I had since become eighty-five pounds heavier. For the next three decades my body weight drifted between 210 and 230 pounds. Except for my knee problems, I seldom had any need to go to a doctor for illness during that time. However, as I was approaching sixty, I had one very physically trying year. During that one year, I made a total of sixty-six visits to either a doctor or a hospital. This was a radical change for me, and I believe this number of medical visits in one year is pretty extravagant for most people. It was a troublesome year, and I was beginning to experience a sense of desperation. I began to wonder if this was just a part of growing older. I wasn't sure.

During this time, I recalled how fit I used to be and wondered if I could recover some of that lost fitness just by making some changes in my lifestyle. I was pretty sure that I needed to lose some weight. I was convinced that I owed it to myself to take some action because doing nothing obviously wasn't working very well. I read many articles and books on the subjects of healthy eating and exercise. While there are many different fitness programs, I combined components from various programs that I believed could work. Based upon my training from my Bachelor of Science degree in health, physical education, and science and my coaching experience, I combined components from various programs that I believed had the proper balance between a healthy eating plan and an adequate exercise program. I decided to implement a program strictly for three months with hopes of positive results. I decided which components to include in the Healthy Vessels program as a result of my previous studies and experiences as well as the results of my twelve-week program.

During my three-month transition I experienced results that were better than I expected. My weight dropped from 224 to 185 pounds. My waistline went from forty inches to thirty-three inches. My blood pressure dropped from 145/95 to 111/61. My pulse rate fell from sixty-five beats per minute to forty-five beats per minute. When I began my program, I had arthritis pain daily at the joint of my left thumb, and I took Vioxx each day to relieve the discomfort. At the end of the program and for the past eight years, I have had no pain in this area. Before I began my nutrition and exercise program, I regularly experienced acid indigestion symptoms, and I took Rolaids and Tums regularly to neutralize the acid. By the end of my three-month challenge, I was taking no antacid medication, and, for more than eight years, I have not had the occasion to do so. Due to a much stronger immune system, I have had no illnesses—not even a common cold or flu—for over eight years. During this same time I have had no doctor visits due to illness. I am now sixty-four years old.

These positive physical changes that I experienced were all that I needed to realize that *what we eat and the activity that we engage in can have very positive personal health benefits.* For me, most of these positive changes took place within just a three-month time period. It was almost unbelievable. I was and still am very thankful that I took the action that I did. It was a small price to pay—changing my eating habits and engaging in regular exercise—for the great benefits that I have received. Now I have a tremendous amount of energy, and I feel extremely fit. My blood pressure is down; my weight is down; my strength is greater; and I have experienced no illnesses during this time. My right knee is stabilized and stronger, and I have a much more positive attitude about my present health. In addition to the positive physical symptoms, I no longer need to be in and out of doctor's offices with the accompanying costs. It is *all good!*

In November of 2008, I met with Pastor Walt Sheppard at Cornerstone Baptist Church in Findlay, Ohio, to inquire about potential areas in the church where I might perform a service of some kind. During that meeting, I mentioned the health program that I had begun in 2002. I showed the pastor some photos that I had taken at the beginning and the end of the three-month program. He indicated an interest in improving his own health and asked me if I could help him. I agreed because I felt it would be a true privilege to help someone receive the health benefits that I was able to receive. Pastor Sheppard was a good student and carefully followed the eating and exercise guidelines that I shared with him.

During the three-month program, Pastor Sheppard lost thirty-seven pounds of undesirable body weight. He went from 224 pounds to a fit 187 pounds at six foot two. Even though he lost a significant amount of weight, he was able to improve his strength during this same time—up to 60 percent in certain exercises. He lost all of the sleep apnea symptoms that he had suffered prior to beginning the program.

Two other church leaders experienced outstanding results as well. Their changes served as an inspiration to others. Pastor Sheppard's former secretary lost more than seventy-five pounds and no longer needed blood pressure medication. Pastor Sheppard's assistant lost forty-five pounds as a result of following the program guidelines. These two church members were examples of how one can make positive health changes in a relatively short period of time and reap great benefits.

It was a true blessing that the three most visible people in our church made such outstanding improvements in their personal health. Because of their great success, they became examples of leadership for the church family. Others have followed their lead. I am now convinced that as you change from an unhealthy lifestyle to a healthy one, you will receive health benefits quickly.

During the time period that I was working with Pastor Sheppard, we discussed the value of developing a twelve-week class to help others at Cornerstone Baptist Church. We believed that unhealthy lifestyles were a problem of both the secular and Christian worlds. With two-thirds of all Americans being either overweight or obese, this is a significant and growing problem in our country. It seemed like a noble venture to give others the tools to combat and neutralize their personal health challenges. I was very confident that the changes that I had made would also produce a positive health impact for others.

With so many prayer requests related to health issues, I believed that it was likely that there were others who were practicing many of the unhealthy habits that I once had. My thinking was that if others could realize some health benefits through a similar program to the one I had put myself and members of the church staff through, it would be a very positive thing. Being sick is not fun, and I believed that if I could make an impact by helping others, it was something I should do. I assumed that there were others who didn't know what to do to improve their health and figured if I could communicate that information to them, there was a good possibility that they would experience improvements in their health. By taking care of their bodies, they would serve as positive Christian examples. There was much to gain and little to lose from my perspective. This was the beginning of my Christian health service.

Pastor Sheppard and I talked about what we would name the class and discussed a number of ideas. My wife, Terri, came up with the name Healthy Vessels. In 1 Thessalonians 4:4 the Bible says, "That every one of you should know how to possess his vessel in sanctification and honour." The word *vessel* in Christian theology has been understood to simply signify a human being. In 1 Thessalonians 4:4, *vessel* may signify either the man's own body or his wife's body. Based upon this meaning it seemed appropriate to make reference to a "healthy vessel" since that is a goal of the Healthy Vessels program. We want to honor God by taking care of the bodies that He has entrusted to us because the Bible tells us to honor God in our bodies. At the end of 2008, we decided to hold three twelve-week sessions for those church members who indicated an interest. Our goal was to limit the first class to fifteen participants. We signed up seventeen church members to launch our first class.

Our first Healthy Vessels class at Cornerstone Baptist Church began in February 2009 and ended in May 2009. I volunteered as the instructor, and my wife agreed to serve in a supportive role. Of the seventeen participants, fifteen were considered overweight, using the body mass index as a point of reference. We lost two class members due to work schedule changes, and three others did not finish the class. I understand that change is difficult and cannot occur unless someone really wants to change. We witnessed excellent results from those who were willing to make changes in their lives.

Our class of twelve lost a total of 286 pounds, with five individuals losing more than 10 percent of their body weight. This does not fully represent the scope of progress that was made because a number of the participants began to work with family members and friends who were not in the class. The reports regarding those individuals have also been very positive. Those in the class who were overweight lost an average of eighteen pounds each, and five individuals lost more than twenty pounds. A number of the class members were on medications at the beginning of our first class, but during our first twelve-week class, our participants were taken off a total of *ten* different medications that had been prescribed by their doctors. Our first twelve-week Healthy Vessels class was a success!

The second Healthy Vessels class began on June 1, 2009, and ended August 24, 2009. The eighteen participants lost almost two hundred pounds. During 2009, those members at Cornerstone Baptist Church who embraced the Healthy Vessels principles in the three classes lost more than seven hundred pounds, and their doctors took them off numerous medications that had previously been prescribed.

From January through April of 2010, my wife and I conducted a twelve-week class in Port Charlotte, Florida, at Tri-City Baptist Church. Class members experienced the same excellent results that we had witnessed at Cornerstone Baptist Church. The class lost more than five hundred pounds and experienced a variety of positive healthy results due to their efforts in following the program.

I realize the importance of leading by example and have made it a priority to do so. Since I began my transformation more than eight years ago, I have continued to incorporate those same principles that turned my life around. I have continued to increase my body strength and have remained free of illness. The principles that I began to follow more than eight years ago as part of a *program* are now part of my *lifestyle*. At age sixty-four, I have been able to accomplish some things that I was not able to do during my most athletic years. I do not consider myself to be a weightlifter, yet I have been able to do better than expected considering my age and experience. This past year I was able to complete 115 consecutive pushups. I recently completed thirty-two consecutive pull-ups. When I was younger, I couldn't even come close to those numbers! I am able to do leg squats with 350 pounds and dead lift 450 pounds. I was never able to dead lift 450 pounds when I was younger. I only mention these examples to illustrate that growing older does not necessarily limit our ability to achieve high levels of fitness.

Prior to developing new lifestyle habits, I would never have believed that this kind of progress was possible at my age. Not only have I made great progress, I have observed the same types of improvements in others who have been willing to make the same fundamental changes that I made. The key to success in achieving good health is to know what to do and then be willing to do it. The "how-to" is the focus of the Healthy Vessels program. The "will do" is the responsibility of the class participants.

It is not difficult to understand what needs to be done to maximize your personal health: you need to eat less and move more. I believe that the Healthy Vessels program can provide a positive benefit in assisting Christians in their desire to reverse some unhealthy habits. The Healthy Vessels program provides guidelines for healthy eating and an exercise plan to support a healthy body weight. This lifestyle program aims at reducing the likelihood of developing a debilitating disease and reducing one's need for dependency upon medication. In addition to attaining a healthy body weight, an equal emphasis is placed upon the importance of cellular nutrition. Our bodies are made up of trillions of tiny cells that are the building blocks of our body. Healthy cells that receive proper nutrition provide us with natural energy, resistance to oxidative stress, and a reduced risk of degenerative diseases. We are really only as healthy as our cells.

During the twelve-week program, approximately thirty to thirty-five hours of instruction are provided. The instructional content was developed from the actual results that I achieved during my initial twelve-week program, my research over the past eight years, my past participation in athletics, and my coaching experience. I have also been able to apply what I used in earning my bachelor of science degree in health, physical education, and science as well as what I am currently learning as a student in Bible college. The class sessions utilize support groups, medical research, guest speakers, class demonstrations, PowerPoint presentations, and use of related video clips.

In our sedentary society, you need to schedule intentional exercise workouts. For those who have no medical limitations, I recommend three to four aerobic workouts and three weight-resistance workouts each week. Portion control and caloric parameters are also essential components to avoiding the accumulation of excessive body weight. Excessive body weight is a high risk factor for many debilitating diseases. It is important to maintain a normal weight as defined by the body mass index. An index reading between 18.5 to 24.9 indicates a normal body weight for a healthy person. Including antioxidant rich foods, five to eight servings of fruits and/or vegetables, and drinking eight to ten eight-ounce glasses of water daily are other important healthy components. When you get enough sleep, eat the right amount of food, make healthy food choices, and exercise properly, you are taking huge strides toward maximizing your health. First Corinthians 6:19–20 says, "What? Know ye not that your body is the temple of the Holy Ghost which is in you, which ye have of God, and ye are not your own? For ye are bought with a price: therefore glorify God in your body, and in your spirit, which are God's." This is good advice for everyone to follow!

Helping others to prevent disease and regain the health that they have lost is a venture based in Christian love. As our overall population continues to become less healthy, are there any clues in the Bible that suggest a direction that Christians should take that will lead them closer to God's will regarding how we should take care of our bodies? Let's look at a Biblical perspective regarding the care we should give to our bodies during our lives on earth.

Chapter 1:

A Biblical Perspective Regarding Your Health

The Bible is clear: God loves us and sent His only begotten Son to die for our sins. The Bible also tells us that God has a perfect will for our lives. God wants all people to be saved, and He desires each one of us to learn to walk in close relationship with Him. A first step is to be obedient to the teachings of Christ. This begins by having faith that God exists and that you have begun a new life in Christ. His will for you can be revealed in a number of ways. The Father will lead you by bringing a verse or a passage of Scripture to your attention. He will use this verse or passage to guide your decisions. You need to ask God to speak to your heart. You may receive an answer quickly, or it might take time before you are ready to hear His voice. God can speak to us through both our opportunities and our obstacles. Wise godly counsel from God's Word can lead you toward God's will. How God reveals His will for each one of us is both unique and personal. But one thing is clear: we are not in God's perfect will when we behave in a manner that contradicts His Word.

Since we are in the church age, we all have a race to run—the Great Commission—while we are alive on this earth. One of our greatest missions is to utilize the gifts and talents that we have been given and make use of them in Christian ministry or Christian service. If we invite illness and disease into our life due to unhealthy habits and practices, we risk our effectiveness to take advantage of the abilities and skills that we have to glorify God. Therefore, it is a good testimony to take care of your body. When you have a desire to demonstrate the power of God working in and through you, taking care of your body could be another way to enhance your personal witness for Christ and bring glory to God. These are appropriate spiritual reasons to take care of your body. You are alive for a purpose!

It is inconsistent with Biblical teaching when you make decisions that hamper your mission. Abusing your body by making decisions that cause your physical body to be compromised will inhibit or diminish your ability to do what God desires for you to do. That would be in direct conflict to God's will for your life.

You should begin by considering whether Christians should look to the Bible for answers regarding health issues. It is my personal belief that the Bible is the ultimate guidebook for living. There is personal application in the Bible for every experience in life. We can learn from direct commandments, from the experiences of people discussed in the Bible, from the life of Jesus, from parables, from the details of others' hardships, and from prophecy. We learn about what types of behaviors in the Bible were blessed and what types of behaviors resulted in negative consequences. Regardless of the behavioral choices that you make, there are consequences. These consequences can be pleasant or unpleasant. I believe there are verses in the Bible that address and guide you to an understanding of what you need to do regarding your health. Second Timothy 3:16–17 tells us that, "All scripture is given by inspiration of God, and is profitable for doctrine, for reproof, for correction, for instruction in righteousness: That the man of God may be perfect, thoroughly furnished unto all good works." This verse is evidence that you can learn from and obtain direction in life by studying scripture.

Because the Bible is clear that you were born with a sinful nature, it is not unusual to accept scriptures and their applications if you like them and then minimize or reject certain other scriptures and their applications because you simply do not want to follow them. This is where many Christians are with the health issue.

Rather than addressing the issue as to how you can best glorify God in your body, it is easy to minimize this verse and scream "Vanity!" because you lack the self-control and discipline to control what you eat and how much you eat. Early in Genesis, God specified the types of food that Adam and Eve should consume. These foods are still healthy choices today.

In the Old Testament Daniel refused to eat the meals provided by King Nebuchadnezzar. Daniel saw a distinction between which foods were proper and which were not. In Daniel 2:8 we read, "But Daniel purposed in his heart that he would not defile himself with the portion of the king's meat, nor with the wine which he drank: therefore he requested of the prince of the eunuchs that he might not defile himself." If there were foods that would defile a Christian in Daniel's time, is it not believable that there are foods today that defile the body? I believe today that we are reaping the consequences of this reality. In Daniel 1:15–16, we see evidence that the diet that Daniel was permitted to follow resulted in a healthier appearance in just ten days. The truth is that what you eat and how much you eat does impact your health.

Proverbs 23:2 is about as direct as a verse can be. It says, "And put a knife to thy throat if thou be a man given to appetite." The application of this verse is that you should control your appetite. Proverbs 23:21 gives another warning: "For the drunkard and the glutton shall come to poverty." This verse makes no distinction between a drunkard and one who overeats. I believe that abuse is abuse. There is no hierarchy when it comes to the abuse of your body. It is no more admirable to abuse your body with food than it is to abuse your body with alcohol. They are both forms of abuse.

Romans 8:8 tells us that "So then they that are in the flesh cannot please God." The abuse of food is a flesh issue. This verse tells us that we cannot please God when our focus is on the flesh. Self-control, a fruit of the Spirit, and discipline are the opposite qualities of living in the flesh. Romans 12:2 instructs Christians that we are to be different from the ways of this world: "And be not conformed to this world: but be ye transformed by the renewing of your mind, that ye may prove what is that good, and acceptable, and perfect, will of God." This verse tells you that you are not supposed to engage in some of the practices that exist in this world.

Daniel took a stand with food. He believed it was important to avoid defiling his body. He apparently believed that certain foods were good for the body and other foods were not. Christians need to set a much higher health standard. We have become careless as a group. This is certainly the case in the area of food. Many Christians eat like the rest of the world and do not appear to have grasped the concept that their bodies are the temples of the Holy Spirit. If the Bible makes reference to your body and food, it is an area that should not be minimized. Should Christians look to the Bible for answers regarding health issues? *Yes!* You can and you should look to the Bible for direction in health issues as well as other issues. When I made some basic, simple changes in my food choices, I went from sixty-six illness-related doctor visits in one year to no illness-related visits for more than eight years. Based upon this dramatic personal experience, I am absolutely convinced that there is a proper and an improper way to eat and drink and that the choices that you make will have much to do with the health of your body.

Consider the fact that obesity is an epidemic in the United States. With more than 67 percent of Americans being either overweight or obese, it is no exaggeration to call it an epidemic. There are volumes of documented studies that identify the accumulation of excess weight as a significant risk factor for a large number of debilitating diseases. It can be challenging enough in this life to do what you should do when your health is good. When you become plagued with medical problems and illnesses, it is much more difficult to keep focused on the task at hand. I experienced this during the year that I had sixty-six medical visits. The Bible is clear that you are to glorify God in your body. When you do glorify God by taking care of your body, you will not make the lifestyle choices that are likely to cause many of the serious health problems that millions of people are experiencing. Taking care of your body is but one way to prevent you from sabotaging God's will or mission for your life.

Despite all of the excuses and rationalizations that exist, the obesity epidemic could not exist without people either eating the wrong foods or eating too much food. To further complicate this problem, a large number of Americans have sedentary lifestyles. First Corinthians 6:19–20 tells Christians that each of our bodies is the temple of the Holy Spirit. It tells us that our bodies are not really our own to do with as we please because we were bought with a price through the death of Christ. We are told that we are to glorify God in our bodies and in our spirits, but it is impossible to glorify God in your body when you abuse it. Unhealthy eating is a form of abuse. Overeating causes an increase in sickness and disease, and obesity is a symptom indicating that you are not taking care of your body.

It is not unusual in the Christian world to be accused of vanity when the issue of taking care of your body is brought up. Personally, when I hear that argument, I believe it is no more than an excuse or rationalization to avoid making the lifestyle decisions that would be more pleasing to God. The Biblical teaching is a simple one: your body is the temple of the Holy Spirit, and it is your responsibility to take care of it! With that said, does the lifestyle that you have adopted conflict with God's plan for your life? Is the core issue of unhealthy choices a spiritual problem?

Spiritually, is it right to want to lose weight? Doesn't God love you unconditionally just the way you are? Is it worldly behavior to focus on wanting to lose weight since spiritual matters are more important than physical ones? Well, consider this: motives are expressions of the heart. It is possible to have wrong motives for just about everything. Let's consider a possible wrong spiritual motive to lose weight. It is possible to desire to lose weight to provoke lust even when it masquerades as a desire to obtain good health. You may want to lose weight just for your personal pride. If the goal is to lose weight for the purpose of getting more attention as a result of a more attractive body, that is a pride issue.

On the opposite end, it is also possible that pride could be the reason that you fail to lose weight. A lack of humility can cause you to fail to exercise the self-control that comes when you yield to the Holy Spirit. It is also possible to become so obsessed with being thin that you can actually compromise your health. Coupled with the constant advertising that you see each day on television and in magazine articles that feature "attractive" men and women, you can desire to conform to these images in a desire to please others. All of these reasons would not be considered appropriate spiritual motives to lose weight.

However, there are some genuinely appropriate motives to lose weight that are consistent with spiritual principles. It is spiritually appropriate and practical to desire to lose weight to improve your health and improve the quality of your life. Having an unhealthy body caused by lifestyle choices is outside of God's perfect will for your life. You are encouraged to take care of your body. A loving God who extends His grace in many areas of your life wants the best for you.

Why We're Overweight

From my observations, I have identified several reasons why so many people allow themselves to become overweight:

1. **Lack of knowledge about food.** Some people may not honestly realize how much they eat, the number of calories that they consume, the nutritional needs of their bodies, or the effect that their eating habits have on their personal health. For these individuals the solution is simply to become informed about how food impacts their bodies. Of course, after knowledge, it is imperative that application of that knowledge follow.

2. **Lack of knowledge about metabolism and movement.** There are things that you can do to increase your body's metabolism. Movement and activity play a huge role in this area. Not understanding the caloric costs of various activities can be a main cause for the negative consequences of overeating. Not only do you need to know about food, you need to know how various activities burn the food that you eat. An active person can eat more calories than an inactive person and avoid

becoming overweight or obese. Once this knowledge is obtained, application of that knowledge is essential.

3. **Lack of knowledge of bad habits.** Sometimes people begin or continue habits, and they do not even realize the impact of their habits. Some examples include eating snacks late in the evening, failing to eat enough fruits and vegetables each day, not drinking enough water each day, consuming too many calories each day, and including too many processed foods in their diets. It is important to take inventory of your eating habits and patterns and learn the impact of them. Failure to understand your habits and patterns will likely have you repeating them mindlessly without realizing the effects on your health.

4. **Spiritual discontent.** When you live a self-centered, self-serving life that is absent from the calling of God you can get in trouble with food. God wants you to get your comfort from Him. When you lack spiritual fulfillment you may attempt to fill that void in many different ways. One of those ways is through food. Philippians 4:13 says, "I can do all things through Christ which strengtheneth me." *All* things would include breaking the bonds of abusing food.

5. **Emotional discontent.** Sometimes your emotional needs are not met, and you may attempt to compensate for this void with other things. When you are unhappy, eating for comfort can be one of the reasons for an overreliance upon food. Boredom and loneliness are two major causes of emotional eating.

6. **Lack of self-control.** Some people have trouble denying themselves. Self-discipline requires that you say no to yourself when it is in your best interest.

Jim Williamson, BS, MA, EdS

The Foods That Were Made for Us to Eat

The first reference to food in the Bible is found in Genesis 1:29. It says, "And God said, Behold, I have given you every herb bearing seed, which is upon the face of all the earth, and every tree, in the which is the fruit of a tree yielding seed; to you it shall be for meat." Is there something to be learned regarding the types of food that the Creator first provided for His creation? Is there any significance that God created fruits, vegetables, grains, beans, nuts, and seeds as our food sources? In the first chapter of Daniel, we learn that Daniel was one of the chosen Israelites brought to King Nebuchadnezzar's palace to learn the culture and language of the Chaldeans. King Nebuchadnezzar's plan was to allow those chosen to partake of the king's diet and of the wine that he drank. It is recorded in Daniel 1:8, "But Daniel purposed in his heart that he would not defile himself with the portion of the king's meat, nor with the wine which he drank: therefore he requested of the prince of the eunuchs that he might not defile himself." Daniel's request was to be allowed to eat vegetables and drink water for ten days instead of the king's eating plan. His request was made to test the impact of his diet as compared to those who ate the diet proposed by the king. Daniel, and his friends Hananiah, Mishael, and Azariah, were given approval for the diet variation. Daniel 1:15–16 tells us that "At the end of ten days their countenances appeared fairer and fatter in flesh than the children which did eat the portion of the king's meat. Thus Melzar took away the portion of their meat, and the wine that they should drink; and gave them pulse (vegetables)." Because of the healthier visual results after just ten days, Daniel was allowed to follow his preferred diet instead of that promoted by the king. The diet that Daniel believed would defile his body was considered inferior. Have we adopted an inferior diet today that is similar to Nebuchadnezzar's diet? It is apparent today that many Christians have accepted a diet that Daniel long ago believed would defile him.

God deliberately created fruits, vegetables, grains, beans, nuts, and seeds for our food sources. If God is perfect, would He not know what is best for the nourishment of our bodies? It seems logical if these were the foods provided during the creation, that these would be the foundational foods which would best meet man's nutritional needs throughout the ages. We first learn in Genesis 9 that God gave mankind permission to eat meat.

There is evidence and support today that these food groups should still be considered vital for good health. The American Cancer Society and other healthy-eating advocates have recommended that fruits and vegetables serve as the foundation of our food choices. For years they have been recommending five to eight servings of fruits and/or vegetables per day to prevent certain diseases.[1] However, accepting *minimum* standards is not necessarily going to lead to *optimal* health. I personally recommend that you eat six to eight servings of fruits and/or vegetables per day. When it comes to fruits and vegetables, I believe more is better!

Does it make sense that the Creator would not know what foods would be best to sustain His creation? Why did Daniel, a devout Israelite, believe that he would be defiling his body if he agreed to eat and drink the diet proposed by the king? There seems to be a close correlation between the foods that King Nebuchadnezzar prescribed and the present American diet. Could it be that many Americans are in fact defiling their own bodies? Are some people rejecting the food choices that God created for our own well-being and replacing healthy foods with inferior food choices? There is evidence that this is happening in America. Though the breadth of the application is not clear, the Bible tells us that God placed some restrictions on what people were to eat. Genesis 2:16–17 says, "And the Lord God commanded the man, saying, of every tree of the garden thou mayest surely eat: but of the tree of the knowledge of good and evil, thou shall not eat of it: for in the day that thou eatest thereof thou shall surely die." This was clearly a command that attached consequences to disobedience.

The Issue of Self-Control

In addition to not eating the appropriate foods, has mankind also become guilty of overindulgence and a lack of self-control? Maybe the same truth applies today as it did in the Garden of Eden. It may be best if you just leave certain foods alone. In 1 Corinthians 6:12, the apostle Paul teaches: "All things are lawful unto me, but all things are not expedient: all things are lawful for me, but I will not be brought under the power of any." This verse reminds us that, although we have the freedom to do many things, we should not allow those things to dominate us. There are times when it is in our best interest to exercise self-control. This verse can be applied to many issues, including—but not limited to—food.

First Corinthians 9:25 says, "And every man that striveth for the mastery is temperate in all things." The word *temperate* means "has self-control." The Bible lists one of the fruits of the Spirit as self-control. The term *fruit of the Spirit* refers to the Holy Spirit that is present in every Christian who accepts Jesus Christ as Lord and Savior. It is God's love and work within and through us. As we mature we are able to bear and convey His fruit. The goal is to build Christlike qualities in our lives so that we can project these qualities onto others. These qualities develop as our relationships with Christ grow through faith in Him. Galatians 5:22–23 identifies qualities that are fruits of the Spirit: "But the fruit of the Spirit is love, joy, peace, longsuffering, gentleness, goodness, faith, meekness, temperance (self-control): against such there is no law."

There is significant evidence that people in America do not exercise self-control in many areas of their lives. Examples may include: a person who makes excessive credit card charges that cause serious financial problems or a person who continues to consume more calories than he can possibly burn off. The evidence is overwhelming that there is a problem with controlling the amount of food that we eat. The growing number of cases of obesity in America testifies to this. Isn't it logical that, if God cares about you and gives you work to complete, He must also care about your physical body and want you to be healthy so you can carry out your mission in life more effectively?

Many people will view weight control as simply a vain activity that parallels the Hollywood, movie-star mind-set. However, the Bible tells us that our bodies are not our own and that we are to glorify God in our bodies. First Corinthians 6:19–20 says, "What? Know ye not that your body is the temple of the Holy Ghost which is in you, which ye have of God, and ye are not your own? For ye are bought with a price: therefore glorify God in your body, and in your spirit, which are God's." This is a command. You are instructed to glorify God in your body and spirit. Is it really possible to abuse food, become obese, and still profess that you are glorifying God in your body? It is impossible to glorify God in the area of health when you do not take care of your body. Becoming obese is a direct contradiction to the goal that we glorify God in our bodies. If the body is the temple of the Holy Spirit, then it is important not to abuse the body. Obesity is an abuse of the body.

The lack of self-control is a dominant characteristic in our society (as evidenced by the obesity epidemic, among other things) and one that the Bible tells us will continue to be so during the last days. Second Timothy 3:1–4 says, "This know also, that in the last days perilous times shall come. For men shall be lovers of their own selves, covetous, boasters, proud, blasphemers, disobedient to parents, unthankful, unholy, without natural affection, trucebreakers, false accusers, incontinent, fierce, despisers of those that are good, traitors heady, high-minded, lovers of pleasures more than lovers of God …" *Incontinent*, in this context, means lacking self-restraint, a quality that can apply to many situations, including the consumption of food. A lack of restraint is a lack of restraint regardless of the application. Self-control is portrayed as a positive quality in the Bible, and a lack of self-control or lack of self-restraint is characterized in a negative light. It should be your personal desire to practice those qualities that are pleasing to God.

The Inner Battle: Flesh versus Spirit

The Bible has many verses that depict the battle between our human flesh and the Spirit. Overeating is a problem with the flesh and lack of control over the flesh. What reinforces and complicates this problem further is that overeating is an acceptable vice in our culture. The Bible tells us that we cannot please God when we live in the flesh.

Romans 8:8 says, "So then they that are in the flesh cannot please God." An overreliance upon the things of the flesh is not a quality that pleases God. Romans 8:5 says, "For they that are after the flesh do mind the things of the flesh; but they that are after the Spirit the things of the Spirit." The Bible is clear that walking in the Spirit is the opposite of following the lead of the flesh.

To further complicate the conflict between the Spirit and the flesh, the Bible reminds us that the flesh is weak. Mark 14:38 says, "Watch ye and pray, lest ye enter into temptation. The spirit is truly ready, but the flesh is weak." This verse reminds you that you are naturally vulnerable to submit to the flesh. Yet you are instructed to live in the Spirit and not the flesh. Galatians 5:16–17 says, "This I say then, walk in the Spirit, and ye shall not fulfill the lust of the flesh. For the flesh lusteth against the Spirit, and the Spirit against the flesh: and these are contrary the one to the other: so that ye cannot do the things that ye would." Romans 8:1 tells you that, "There is therefore now no condemnation to them which are in Christ Jesus who walk not after the flesh, but after the Spirit." The habit of overeating occurs when the flesh desires more than a healthy portion of food. You are commanded not to walk after the flesh. Food was created to sustain life on earth. You should eat to live. When people began "living to eat," they started making the decision to expand the role of food in their lives beyond what was intended.

The Bible warns you that Satan, our enemy, is a tempter for all who live in the flesh rather than the Spirit. First Peter 5:8 warns, "Be sober, be vigilant; because your adversary the devil, as a roaring lion, walketh about, seeking whom he may devour." Satan is not the fictitious creature that is often depicted in the media. In Genesis 3:1 you read about the manipulative potential of Satan. This verse says, "Now the serpent (Satan) was more subtle than any beast of the field which the Lord God had made." To provide evidence of Satan's effectiveness, Scripture gives us a description of the behaviors that are prominent in a world outside of Christ. First John 1:16 says, "For all that is in the world, the lust of the flesh, and the lust of the eyes, and the pride of life, is not of the father, but is of the world." We also learn from Scripture that those outside of Christ see nothing particularly wrong with living in the flesh. First Corinthians 2:14 says, "But the natural man receiveth not the things of the Spirit of God: for they are foolishness unto him: neither can he know them, because they are spiritually discerned."

Is there any remedy that can aid us in combating the flesh? The Bible tells us that we are in a battle with an enemy that is not visible with the human eye. Ephesians 6:11–13 advises, "Put on the whole armour of God, that ye may be able to stand against the wiles of the devil. For we wrestle not against flesh and blood, but against principalities, against powers, against the rulers of the darkness of this world, against spiritual wickedness in high places. Wherefore take unto you the whole armour of God, that ye may be able to withstand in the evil day, and having done all, to stand." A first step is to realize that you are in the midst of a spiritual battle in which Satan wants to destroy you. It would be his desire to destroy your family, your faith, your testimony, your hope, and your health. It is difficult for you to defend yourself if you are not even aware that a battle is taking place. That is why you are told to be sober and vigilant. It is not beneath Satan to influence you with certain habits that would destroy your health so that you cannot live out God's perfect will for your life. Poor health can be a powerful contributor to discouragement and depression.

In James 4:7 we receive this message: "Submit yourselves therefore to God. Resist the devil, and he will flee from you." If you are a follower of Christ, you can overcome the temptations of this world and the unhealthy habits that are practiced by the masses. Being a follower of Christ requires a mind-set and focus that are different from what is typical in this world. We are to be led by the Spirit and not by the ways of this world. Though we cannot be perfect, our efforts should be directed toward living in a manner that is pleasing to God.

What the Bible Says about Consequences

Are there consequences when we fail to leave certain foods alone or fail to exercise self-control in our eating and drinking? Since God has a perfect will for each of our lives, it makes sense that we may be inhibited in our missions if we do those things that result in self-inflicted sicknesses or disabilities. When we do things that disrupt our missions, does that matter to God? The Bible tells us that when we are disobedient, there are consequences. Galatians 6:7–8 says, "Be not deceived; God is not mocked: for whatsoever a man soweth, that shall he also reap. For he that soweth to his flesh shall of the flesh reap corruption; but he that soweth to the Spirit shall of the Spirit reap life everlasting."

There are consequences when you allow your flesh to disobey God's Word. You need to exercise self-control in the area of food, as in other areas. When you fail to exercise self-control, you are inviting undesirable consequences.

One of the biggest problems in our society regarding food is that overeating and abuse of food is not seen as a serious problem even though the financial and personal health costs prove that it is. Too often, overeating is seen as an acceptable vice. Even so, it is a vice that invites undesirable consequences.

Does the Bible have a view about overeating? Proverbs 23:21 says, "For the drunkard and the glutton shall come to poverty." One definition of a glutton is one who overeats. In this passage, the Bible reference does not portray overeating as a desirable trait. While most Christians understand that drunkenness is not God's will, there is a tendency to minimize the problem with gluttony. Proverbs 23:2 says, "And put a knife to thy throat, if thou be a man given to appetite." This verse is pretty direct in presenting overeating as a negative quality.

Those who are eating and drinking in an unhealthy manner are the people who are suffering the most from debilitating diseases. Heart disease is the number one cause of death in America, and cancer is the number two cause of death. There is a definite link between food and lifestyle choices for both of these diseases. It is not a coincidence that Americans have a greater incidence of these diseases when compared to people in many other countries. Poor eating habits are causing many to become weak and sickly and many die prematurely; eating in an unworthy manner is a major cause of obesity, and obesity is a serious health risk factor that results in a greater risk for many other debilitating diseases.

Obesity-related illnesses are responsible for a large number of deaths each year. The CDC (Centers for Disease Control) has adopted a new way of recording these deaths. In 2004, they issued an annual estimate of 365,000 obesity related deaths, and the next year they estimated that 112,000 American deaths were obesity related.[2] This decrease in deaths is not a sign that obesity has become less deadly. Instead, the change in numbers reflects a change in the recording methods that are used to report the data. There are, however, a number of sources that continue to estimate obesity related deaths at three hundred thousand or more each year including those within the CDC.[3] There is a serious problem in accurately reporting these deaths. For example, if I were two hundred pounds overweight and died from a heart attack, that statistic could be reported two ways. One way is to report that I died from a heart attack. The second way to report this death would be to say that the heart attack was obesity related. I would be more inclined to report this death as obesity related rather than merely as a heart attack. In this example, obesity would have been a significant factor. Because of the ease with which these statistics can be manipulated, I am inclined to believe that obesity-related deaths far exceed the 112,000 figure identified using the new reporting guidelines. The new way of reporting the data can easily distort reality.

Overeating is presently costing billions of dollars in preventable medical expenses that threaten our health care system and add to the personal misery of millions of individuals. Obesity is now recognized as the number one health problem in America, yet obesity is a preventable disease for those who practice healthy eating.

Why the Church Should Get Involved

There are many problems with the flesh (lust, materialism, being power hungry); food abuse should not be omitted from that list because it is indeed a problem. Some research studies have concluded that 85 percent of all debilitating diseases are caused by unhealthy lifestyle choices. If that percentage is even remotely close to being accurate, then a large number of the health issues suffered by people in the church are preventable. Due to the large number of individuals being impacted by health issues, shouldn't we Christians take a more serious look at what is happening within our own congregations? Instead of promoting church events that feature large amounts of unhealthy foods, it is time for churches to take a serious inventory from within and make some intentional, healthy changes. Reinforcing unhealthy practices is not in the best interest of a Christian congregation. This may not be popular with some people, but it may be the wise thing to do. If Christians are really the "light of the world" (Matthew 5:14), maybe we should assume a leadership role in this area.

Traditionally, in the church setting, there is more enthusiasm for discussing drug abuse, alcohol abuse, and pornography than for addressing food abuse. Food abuse simply is minimized when compared to other forms of abuse even though all forms of abuse are harmful to the body and spirit. It is very tempting to make the argument that the health of our bodies is not as important as other areas that the Bible teaches about. But it is dangerous for us to make arbitrary decisions as to which verses are important based on our feelings. When we make arbitrary decisions, we are picking and choosing. However, if you believe the Bible, you must conclude that God has a purpose when He says that we are to glorify God in our bodies. We should not minimize the importance of any verse in the Bible.

Proverbs 3:5–8 says, "Trust in the Lord with all thine heart; and lean not unto thine own understanding. In all thy ways acknowledge Him, and He shall direct thy paths. Be not wise in thine own eyes: fear the Lord, and depart from evil. It shall be health to thy navel, and marrow to thy bones." This verse reinforces the view that the Bible supplies us with the wisdom that when applied in our lives will maximize our ability to follow the perfect will of God.

Your personal health has much to do with the manner in which you utilize the food that is available. When you knowingly overindulge, you have made a decision not to exercise self-control.

This behavior is an act of disobedience for which there are personal consequences. Out of respect for your loving and holy God, your goal as a Christian should be to practice obedience in all areas of life. You also need to be mindful that failure to practice obedience always has consequences.

What about those people who have compromised their health by practicing unhealthy habits? Can they recover some of the ground they have lost? I cannot promise or predict what is possible for every individual who has compromised his or her health in the past. But I *can* say that I was able to recover much of the health that I had lost due to my previous unhealthy lifestyle choices. I have witnessed others who have been able to improve their health by changing some of their lifestyle choices. I believe that if you do the right thing long enough, something good is likely to happen. This is the faith that I have. Until you are willing to make the changes, you can never know how those changes may impact your health. What do you have to lose? Absolutely nothing! Philippians 4:13 boldly proclaims, "I can do all things through Christ which strengtheneth me."

Chapter 2:

What's The Big Deal?

In order to determine whether there is a health crisis in America, it is important to review the data that is available to us. What is a crisis? Webster's online dictionary defines a *crisis* as an unstable situation of extreme danger or difficulty. The American Heritage dictionary defines a *crisis* as an unstable condition that involves a sudden change toward either improvement or deterioration. Let's examine some health data to see if we can better understand America's current health status.

The Problem of Being Overweight

There have been many warnings and concerns from past and current surgeons general of the United States, the leaders on matters of public health in the U.S. government. C. Everett Koop became surgeon general in 1981 under President Ronald Reagan and soon thereafter warned that the statistics regarding obesity in the United States were "over the top" when compared to other industrialized nations. At that time, approximately 15.5 percent of our youth were considered severely overweight, and an additional 10 percent of youth were "at risk" for becoming overweight. (A person is considered to be severely overweight when he or she has a body mass index over 35.0.)

Koop pointed out the growing trend of young people beginning to experience higher rates of so-called adult diseases such as diabetes and hypertension. He believed the cause of the problem was consumption of *too much food* in relation to their physical activity. He encouraged parents to be role models to their children by demonstrating healthy eating and exercise behaviors. In his opinion, Americans of all ages were starving—not from *lack* of food, as with people in many other countries, but rather from malnourishment due to not eating the proper foods.[1] This unhealthy trend has led to an increase in premature deaths from coronary heart disease, stroke, arteriosclerosis, diabetes, and some kinds of cancer. These debilitating diseases account for more than two-thirds of all deaths in the United States.

On July 16, 2003, Surgeon General Richard Carmona issued a report entitled "The Crisis Is Obesity." In his report to the U.S. House of Representatives, he stated that obesity, which is completely preventable, was the fastest-growing cause of disease and death in America. He noted that two out of three Americans were either overweight or obese and that one out of every eight deaths was caused by an illness directly related to being overweight or obese. Dr. Carmona echoed former Surgeon General Koop by saying that these growing statistics were the direct result of unhealthy eating habits and decreased physical activity. He outlined three key factors that he believed had to be addressed to reduce or eliminate childhood obesity in America: increased physical activity; healthier eating habits, and improved health literacy. Dr. Carmona publicly stated that he believed obesity was the number one health issue in the United States.[2]

In October of 2007 Dr. Steven K. Galson began serving as surgeon general. Consistent with past surgeons general, Dr. Galson expressed his concern about the health of Americans. He noted that there were then 12.5 million overweight children and teens in the United States. Dr. Galson blamed obesity on the increase in food portion sizes while Americans continue to adopt more sedentary lifestyles. He said, "Our children are growing up with unhealthy lifestyles, the consequences of which could be with them for the rest of their lives." He blamed unhealthy lifestyles as the root cause of such childhood health problems as high cholesterol, type 2 diabetes, and asthma. Dr. Galson further reported that chronic diseases cause seven out of ten deaths with staggering financial and physical implications.[3]

Quite simply, Americans were (and are) eating too many foods that are full of empty calories and foods that have high glycemic indexes. These food choices are contributing to making many Americans fat. Foods with high glycemic indexes (over 70) are carbohydrates that break down quickly, resulting in a rapid rise in blood sugar levels. These high glycemic foods dominate the diet of many Americans, and one of the effects of the rise in blood sugar levels associated with these foods is that the excess blood sugar is converted into fat and stored in fat cells. This causes weight gain. The remedy is obvious: we need to reduce overeating, increase activity levels, and eat the right foods.

The Prevalence of Weight Problems

The cost of health care in the United States amounts to more than 13 percent of our gross domestic product (GDP) or nearly $5,000 per capita each year. In spite of past warnings from our Surgeons General and the voices of many others in the healthcare industry, the problem continues to grow. It is a widely held belief that unhealthy lifestyle choices are responsible for up to 85 percent of chronic debilitating diseases. The current health crisis costs approximately $117 billion per year, a figure which includes direct costs like preventive, diagnostic, and treatment services related to weight, as well as indirect costs like absenteeism and loss of future earnings due to premature death. We are currently spending $238 billion a year on obesity-related expenses. It is estimated that we could cut $147 billion out of our health budget if people would just take care of themselves.[4]

Clearly, we are not making progress in making wise choices concerning our health habits, and our current situation can properly be called a national health crisis and an epidemic. Although we spend more money on medical expenses and prevention campaigns than any other country, American obesity rates are the highest in the world. Consider these facts:

1. From 1986 to 2000, we have experienced increases in obesity rates, from one in two hundred adults to one in fifty adults.[5]

2. The rate of extreme obesity has gone from one in two thousand American adults to one in four hundred.[6]

3. Approximately nine million American children six years and older are considered obese.[7]

4. Twenty percent of four-year-old children are considered obese.[8]

5. Every year, between three thousand and five thousand service members are forced to leave the military for being too fat.[9]

6. More than twenty-three million Americans currently have diabetes, nearly 8 percent of the population. Another fifty-seven million adults have blood sugar levels that indicate they are at serious risk of developing diabetes, which is a major cause of kidney failure, stroke, heart disease, lower-limb amputations, and blindness.[10]

7. The Centers for Disease Control estimated that there have been 365,000 obesity-related deaths in 2004. (They have since adopted a new reporting method.)[11]

8. According to a recent analysis from the Research Triangle Institute, the total medical cost of obesity in the United States is $147 billion per year.[12]

9. Being obese increases your risk of suffering from diabetes, heart disease, stroke, arthritis, and some cancers. If you are obese, losing even 5 to 10 percent of your weight can delay or prevent some of these diseases.[13]

10. In 2009, not a single state met the *Healthy People 2010* obesity target of 15 percent. Only Colorado and the District of Columbia had a prevalence of obesity that was less than 20 percent. Thirty-three states had a prevalence of obesity equal to or greater than 25 percent; nine of

these states (Alabama, Arkansas, Kentucky, Louisiana, Mississippi, Missouri, Oklahoma, Tennessee, and West Virginia) had a prevalence of obesity equal to or greater than 30 percent.[14]

11. In 2008 the prevalence of obesity in the United States was 32.2 percent for adult men and 35.5 percent for adult women.[15]

12. Encouraging kids to eat more fruits and vegetables and consume fewer sodas and high-calorie, high-fat snack foods is an essential step in combating childhood obesity. It is also recommended that children engage in about sixty minutes of physical activity each day to combat obesity.[16]

13. The youth of today are becoming heavier at an alarming rate, with nearly 12 million children and adolescents ages two to nineteen considered obese. As these children grow older, they have a much greater risk of developing and dying from chronic diseases in adulthood.[17]

Some people have become too dependent upon our healthcare system. In the 1700s, Benjamin Franklin was quoted as saying, "An ounce of prevention is worth a pound of cure." However, more than two hundred years later, prevention is still a radical concept to many Americans. Why do we treat our automobiles better than we do our own bodies? We make sure that our cars get the right kind of oil, gasoline, engine repairs, and maintenance; yet many people abuse their bodies, and when their bodies break down, they quickly run to a doctor or hospital to secure some sort of medication or surgery. There is no doubt that medication and surgery may be required at times, but much too often these medical options could have been avoided if we had just led healthier lifestyles.

It is clear that personal lifestyle is a major factor in causing chronic diseases. Because of irregularities in reporting, it is difficult to get an accurate assessment of how many chronic diseases are caused by lifestyle choices. I have seen statistical quotes that attribute chronic diseases to lifestyle choices that range between 60 and

85 percent. Whatever the exact figure, it is clear that lifestyle is becoming a more significant factor each year in causing premature death and disease. Diseases such as heart disease, cancer, stroke, diabetes, and hypertension are typically associated with poor lifestyle choices. Epidemic rises in obesity have also created additional health problems.

Dr. Tim Armstrong from the World Health Organization Department of Chronic Diseases and Health Promotion believes that a healthy lifestyle makes a significant difference in whether a person will contact a noncommunicable disease. Diseases such as cancer, cardiovascular disease, and diabetes account for 60 percent of all deaths. These diseases have common risk factors: tobacco use, inappropriate diet, and physical inactivity. It is believed that by avoiding these risk factors in the first place, we can prevent the majority of deaths caused by these diseases. Dr. Armstrong noted that the incidence of colon cancer can be reduced by up to 50 percent by increasing fruit and vegetable consumption.[18] Lifestyle choices are significant factors that help people become healthier which is why lifestyle choices are the focus of the Healthy Vessels program. Small changes can result in big differences!

The World Health Organization (WHO) studied the health systems of 191 countries and reported the findings in the *World Health Report* in 2000. The findings in this report include:

1. The United States spent a higher percentage of its gross domestic product on its health system than any other country.
2. The U.S. health system ranked seventy-second when measuring the performance of health systems, including efficiency.
3. The United States ranked fifty-fifth in fairness of financial contribution toward health care.[19]

Americans too often believe that doctors and prescription medicine are the silver bullets that will turn their personal health crisis around. However, drugs, surgery, and hospitals are rarely the answer to chronic health problems. The majority of Americans continue to believe that if a drug is approved by the Food and Drug Administration (FDA) and prescribed by their doctors, that drug is safe.

Take the case of Vioxx, a drug that belongs to a class of drugs called non-steroidal anti-inflammatory drugs (NSAIDS). It was manufactured and marketed by the pharmaceutical company Merck & Co. from 1999 to 2004. Merck issued a news release in 2003 that acknowledged the use of Vioxx increased the risk of heart problems, including heart attacks and stroke. In 2004, Merck voluntarily decided to pull Vioxx from the market. By then, the drug had been used by more than 84 million people. Up to 50,000 personal injury lawsuits from Vioxx users followed who suffered heart attacks or stroke. In 2007, Merck & Co. agreed to pay $4.8 billion to end thousands of state and federal lawsuits.

Even after Vioxx, we still believe that drugs approved by the FDA must be safe! Some people believe the FDA has a record of providing for fast-track drug approvals—long before there is any solid evidence of possible long-term risks. While a majority of the drugs approved are known to cause some potentially serious side effects in some people—even death—they are approved anyway. There is an assumption that doctors will educate themselves on the drugs they prescribe and monitor their patients to ensure safety. Too often, this does not happen. Studies have shown that doctors rely on pharmaceutical company sales representatives to educate them on drugs, and the FDA relies on pharmaceutical company personnel in the approval process for those drugs. This is a serious conflict of interest with negative effects on public health. Could it be that the interests of the pharmaceutical companies are a higher priority than the welfare of the people?

Our healthcare system continues to spiral downward even though we spend more than $2.3 trillion per year (2008 figure) on our health. This is more than $7,650 per person. Health expenditures in 2008 were 16.2 percent of our gross domestic product (GDP).[20] Maintaining healthy lifestyles is the better, cheaper, and less dangerous alternative for our health.

Beginning in 1950, the amount of nutritional information available to the public has roughly doubled every seven years. Yet during this same period of time, the obesity rate in the United States has grown by more than 200 percent.[21] The amount of information available is not the problem. It has become very obvious that there is not necessarily a relationship between individual behavior and the amount of information available. The most important component contributing to change is the *desire* to change. The catalyst for change is dependent upon a person's capacity to develop a strong enough "why" to make the change. When a strong reason is absent, change is unlikely.

The measure that is most widely used today to assess the healthiness of human body weight is called the body mass index (BMI), which compares a person's weight with their height. Body mass index is not intended as a medical diagnosis but rather a numerical gauge of how much an individual's body weight corresponds to what is considered normal or desirable for a specific height. It is a helpful tool in evaluating your personal health because adverse health risk factors increase in probability when your body weight exceeds the normal weight for your height.[22]

The body mass index is defined as the individual's body weight divided by the square of one's height. These numeric measures are provided on a chart where heights are posted vertically and body weights horizontally (See the body mass index table in the appendix). As you match your height and body weight on the chart, your body mass index is revealed across the top of the chart. Everyone will fall into one of seven classes:

Class	Body Mass Index
Severely underweight	Under 16.5
Underweight	16.5–18.4
Normal weight	18.5–24.9
Overweight	25.0–29.9
Obese	30.0–34.9
Clinically obese	35.0–39.9
Morbidly obese	40.0 and over

By reviewing the following health data as it relates to the body mass index, we get a clearer picture regarding America's growing obesity problem. Though our country spends millions of dollars on obesity prevention, the chart below does not suggest that a positive impact is being realized. The percentage of Americans that are overweight, obese, and severely obese has increased in every one of the six reporting periods from 1950 through 2008 (as data was available). Even as the information regarding the health risks of being overweight becomes more available to the public and the expenditures to fight obesity increase, the number of Americans becoming overweight and obese is also increasing. So far the campaign to reduce the health risk of obesity is failing.

Years	% Overweight	% Obese	% Severe Obesity
1950–1960	33.0	9.7	No Data Available
1964–1970	39.5	11.3	No Data Available
1976–1980	46.0	14.4	No Data Available
1988–1994	56.0	23.	2.9
1999–2000	64.5	30.5	4.7
2008	67.0	33.0	6.0

The Better Option:
Prevention versus Treatment

So how can we overcome our present health crisis? We must address the three areas that were outlined by Surgeon General Carmona in his 2003 report to the House of Representatives, "The Crisis Is Obesity." In subsequent chapters, we will examine the practical solutions to each of Dr. Carmona's three main points:

1. **Increase physical activity.** For important health benefits, adults need at least 150 minutes of moderate intensity aerobic activity (for example, brisk walking) and muscle-strengthening activities on two or more days

a week that work all major muscle groups (legs, hips, back, abdomen, chest, shoulders and arms).[23] Many people simply do not move enough in the sedentary society in which they live. Modern technologies have made tasks easier so that less physical effort is required. We have also eliminated playing, running, and jumping for text messaging, watching television, and spending endless hours on the computer.

2. **Develop healthier eating habits.** A healthy diet emphasizes fruits, vegetables, whole grains, and fat-free or low-fat milk products. It should also include lean meats, poultry, beans, eggs, and nuts. These foods should be low in saturated fats, trans fats, cholesterol, salt (sodium), and added sugars.[24] We need to avoid eating a lot of refined and processed food, such as white rice, TV dinners, cereals, white bread, and products with sugar. We should depend more on nature's best—fruits and vegetables. All food is not equal. Some foods nourish the trillions of cells in our body quite well, and some foods provide little or no nutrition.

3. **Become more health literate.** Too few people understand food labels and the implications of what foods contain. Americans must develop a greater awareness of our health needs and make beneficial choices that impact and help create healthy bodies. There is a tremendous amount of health information available to the general public. Books, magazine articles, the Internet, experts, and television programs provide excellent health information. Those who are lacking the information needed to develop a healthy lifestyle need only to learn healthy principles and then implement them in their lives.

Chapter 3:

A Picture of Health

As the gauges in your automobile tell you how the automobile's systems are operating, body numbers reveal the efficiency of your body. You can also use them to compare your progress toward your goal of becoming a healthier human being. Some of the most significant body numbers used to measure progress in improving health include: blood pressure, heart rate, cholesterol levels, prostate-specific antigen levels (for men), body weight, body mass index, and abdominal size. This chapter provides information that you should know and understand about your body numbers.

Blood Pressure

Your blood pressure is one of the most important body numbers you should be aware of because a high blood pressure reading can cause a number of debilitating conditions and/or death. And, unless blood pressure is checked regularly, it is not always apparent when blood pressure is at a dangerous level.

What is blood pressure? Blood pressure is the force of your blood pushing against your artery walls. Each time your heart beats, it pumps blood out into your arteries. Your blood pressure is the highest when your heart beats, pumping the blood. This pressure is represented by the top number in your blood pressure reading and is called the systolic pressure. For example, if your blood pressure were

118/72, 118 would be your systolic pressure. When your heart is at rest, between beats, your blood pressure is the lowest. This pressure is represented by the bottom number in your blood pressure reading and is called the diastolic pressure. In the above example of 118/72, the bottom number, 72, would be your diastolic pressure.

Healthy Blood Pressure Levels

Blood pressure changes throughout the day. It is lowest when you sleep and higher when you are awake. During most of your waking hours, your blood pressure stays pretty much the same. It can increase when you get excited or nervous or when you are active. When a person is diagnosed with high blood pressure it doesn't mean that a person is too stressed or nervous. This is a popular myth. Many people who are perfectly calm have high blood pressure. The effects of long-term stress on blood pressure are not clearly understood. During short-term stressful situations, stress can make blood pressure increase, but once the stress is relieved, the blood pressure readings return to normal.

An ideal or healthy blood pressure without medication is 115/76.[1] The national median in the United States is 129/86.[2] A blood pressure reading of 140/90 or more is considered high blood pressure. Many doctors believe that your blood pressure should be lower than 120/80. You should be aware of the four levels of blood pressure.

1. Normal blood pressure: Less than 120/80
2. Prehypertension: 120/80 to 139/89
3. Stage 1 high blood pressure: 140/90 to 159/99
4. Stage 2 high blood pressure:= 160/100 or higher[3]

The different stages of high blood pressure usually impact the treatment that is prescribed. Treatment for Stage 1 high blood pressure may depend on certain lifestyle factors. Doctors may choose to immediately begin treatment with medicine or they may allow for a grace period during which the patient is instructed to make certain diet and activity changes in an attempt to reduce their blood pressure naturally. Treatment guidelines allow for much less flexibility with Stage 2 high blood pressure. Those diagnosed at this stage are almost universally given anti-hypertension medicine immediately. Stage 2 high blood pressure also requires more frequent blood pressure checks and more careful monitoring.

The Dangers of High Blood Pressure

High blood pressure can result in a number of unhealthy conditions. It can quietly damage your body for years before symptoms develop. Left uncontrolled, you may wind up with a disability, a poor quality of life, or even a fatal heart attack. Some of the unhealthy conditions are discussed below:

- **Arteriosclerosis and aneurysms.** Excessive pressure in your arteries from high blood pressure alters the cells of the inner lining of the arteries. This condition can make the artery walls thick and stiff, leading to a disease called arteriosclerosis. Over time, the constant pressure of blood through a weakened artery can cause a section of its wall to enlarge and form a bulge. This bulge is called an aneurysm. An aneurysm can rupture and cause life-threatening bleeding to occur in any artery in the body, but the most common area for an aneurysm to occur is in the aorta, the largest artery in the body.[4] The aorta originates from the left ventricle of the heart and extends down to the abdomen, where it branches off into smaller arteries.
- **Heart attacks.** When the left ventricle of the heart contracts, it pushes blood into the aorta; this blood then travels to all the body tissues down to the capillary level. High blood pressure forces your heart to overexert itself, causing the left ventricle to enlarge. This enlargement limits the ventricle's ability to expand sufficiently and to completely fill with blood.[5] This condition increases

the risk of a heart attack, heart failure, or sudden cardiac death. Heart failure occurs when the added exertion demanded by high blood pressure causes your heart to weaken and work less efficiently. Eventually, an overworked heart simply begins to wear out and fail.

- **Transient ischemic attacks (TIAs).** High blood pressure damages and weakens your brain's blood vessels, causing them to narrow, rupture, or leak. A transient ischemic attack (TIA) is a brief, temporary obstruction of the blood supply to your brain. This condition is often referred to as a mini-stroke. It is often caused by a blood clot and should serve as a warning that you are at risk for a full-blown stroke.[6] A stroke occurs when part of your brain is deprived of oxygen and nutrients, causing brain cells to die.

- **Dementia.** Dementia is a brain condition, resulting in impaired thinking, speaking, memory, vision and movement. It can result from the narrowing and blockage of the arteries that supply blood to the brain or occur as a result of a stroke.[7]

- **Mild cognitive impairment.** Mild cognitive impairment is a transition stage between the cognitive changes of normal aging and the more serious problems caused by Alzheimer's disease. This impairment can be linked to damaged arteries from high blood pressure, which inhibits the blood flow to the brain.[8]

- **Kidney failure.** High blood pressure is one of the most common causes of kidney failure. It can damage both of the large arteries leading to the kidneys as well as the tiny blood vessels within the kidneys. Damage to either of these large arteries disrupts your kidneys' ability to filter waste products from your blood.[9] This can lead to your need for either dialysis or kidney transplantation—both serious treatments. The tiny clusters of blood vessels within your kidneys are called glomeruli. These blood vessels filter fluid, waste, and other substances from your blood. A number of different diseases can result in damage to the glomeruli. These diseases can cause swelling or scarring, which can leave your kidneys unable to filter waste effectively, ultimately leading to kidney failure.[10]

A kidney artery aneurism is a bulge in the wall of an artery leading to the kidney. The danger of this condition is that over time, it can rupture and cause life-threatening internal bleeding.[11]

- **Vision impairment.** High blood pressure can damage the vessels supplying blood to the retina in the eye. When damaged, the blood vessels can leak or become blocked. This condition can lead to bleeding in the eye, swelling of the optic nerve, blurred vision, and even a complete loss of eyesight. When you have diabetes with high blood pressure, the risk is even greater. There could also be fluid buildup under the retina, caused by a leaky blood vessel located under the retina, which results in vision distortion and in some cases, scarring that impairs vision.[12] Nerve damage can occur when a blockage of blood flow damages the optic nerve. This condition can lead to dysfunction of the optic nerve cells, which may cause bleeding within your eye. Total vision loss and even death can also occur.[13]

- **Bone loss.** An unhealthy blood pressure may increase the amount of calcium that is eliminated in the urine; that, in turn, may lead to osteoporosis (loss of bone mineral density), increasing the risk for fractures. This risk is especially prominent in elderly women.[14]

- **Sleep apnea.** Many health professionals believe that high blood pressure triggers sleep apnea. Sleep apnea occurs in more than 50 percent of those with high blood pressure.[15] Obstructive sleep apnea reduces the quality of your evening sleep. Because the quality of your sleep is compromised, sleep deprivation can also occur and can further increase blood pressure.

Preventing High Blood Pressure

As is true with most preventable health problems, prevention of circulatory problems is the cure. A sound program that includes the following components will be the best strategy for preventing most of the conditions mentioned above:

1. A healthy eating program that supports maintenance of a body weight in the normal body mass index range and that provides your body with the optimal nutrients that it needs to operate efficiently and effectively. This includes drinking eight to ten eight-ounce glasses of water each day.
2. A well-balanced exercise program that includes both aerobic and weight-resistance exercises.
3. Prioritizing getting an adequate amount of sleep (seven to eight hours) each evening.

Regular aerobic physical activity increases your fitness level and capacity for exercise. It also plays a role in both primary and secondary prevention of cardiovascular disease. Regular physical activity can help control blood lipid abnormalities, diabetes, and obesity. Aerobic physical activity can also help reduce blood pressure. The results of pooled studies show that people who modify their behavior and start regular physical activity after a heart attack have better rates of survival and a better quality of life. Healthy people—as well as many patients with cardiovascular disease—can improve their fitness and exercise performance with training.[16]

Even if you have high blood pressure, there are many benefits of resistance training. Resistance training has been proven to lower diastolic blood pressure. It can help to improve the flexibility of your joints and muscles and ease the strain of exercise, which is a common excuse for not exercising in the first place. Stretching your muscles is also a great stress reliever. Stretching helps people who have stress-induced hypertension. As the muscles strengthen and grow, capillary density increases. This density helps reduce peripheral resistance. Stress hormones are also lowered, which may reduce your blood pressure.[17]

There are significant benefits to both aerobic and weight-resistance exercises, but it is important that you always follow the advice of your physician regarding any limitations that force you to restrict physical activity at the onset. The goal is always to start at a level that is consistent with your current fitness and then build from that point. You should never train beyond your fitness level.

Heart Rate

Your heart rate is measured by the number of times your heart beats in a minute. The average person has a heart rate of sixty to eighty beats per minute.[18] The heart rate of athletes can go as low as forty to sixty beats per minute. An elite athletic heart rate may be even lower than forty beats per minute. An infant's heart rate ranges between 100 and 160 beats per minute.[19]

There are a number of factors that can influence your heart rate. Some of these factors are your age, gender, and physical activity level. A condition referred to as an athlete's heart is a medical syndrome in which the human heart is enlarged due to excessive amounts of exercise. This is a common condition in athletes and in weight trainers who exercise more than an hour every day. A person with athletic heart syndrome has a heart that is larger than normal, and the walls of his or her heart are thicker. The chambers inside the heart are also larger. This increase in size and thickening of the walls allows the heart to pump substantially more blood per heartbeat without an increase in heart rate. This larger volume of blood flowing through the heart results in a slower but stronger pulse. This stronger pulse is sometimes diagnosed as a heart murmur. These murmurs, which are specific sounds created as blood flows through the valves of the heart, are perfectly normal in an athlete and are not dangerous. Athletic heart syndrome is not thought to affect health in any way. The rare sudden deaths of athletes are usually due to underlying heart diseases that were not previously detected rather than to any dangers resulting from athletic heart syndrome.[20]

It can be expected that competitive distance runners, swimmers, cyclists, and other endurance athletes will have lower resting heart rates due to the strength of their hearts. This strength can be attributed to the increase in the size of their hearts that results from training. For example, when I was running cross country in college, my heart rate was thirty-six beats per minute. Miguel Indurain, a cyclist and five-time Tour de France winner, had a resting heart rate of twenty-eight beats per minute. This was one of the lowest resting heart rates ever recorded. It is always the goal of an endurance athlete to have a strong, healthy heart. A lower heart rate from athletic training is evidence of a strong athletic heart.

There are several terms that you should be familiar with when training your body. These include:

1. **Resting Heart Rate.** This is your heart rate at rest. The best time to determine your resting heart rate is in the morning, after a good night's sleep and before you get out of bed. The heart beats about sixty to eighty times a minute when you are at rest. Resting heart rate usually increases with age and is generally lower in physically fit people. The heart rate adapts to changes in your body's need for oxygen, such as during exercise or sleep.

   Try this experiment: While in a resting position, measure your heart rate and see if, by relaxing more and more, you can get your heart rate to drop further. Let's say you might have a heart rate of sixty-three when you start; after a few minutes, it may drop down to fifty-nine or sixty. Once your heart rate has stabilized to a point about as low as it is going to go, you can experiment with small movements and see what changes occur in your heart rate. There is no set goal here, you're just trying to experience what relaxation does to your heart rate and how sensitive your heart rate is to any movement you might make.[21]

2. **Maximum Heart Rate.** This rate refers to the highest number of times a healthy heart should beat during

maximum physical exertion without risking danger. The most common accepted formula is to subtract your age from 220.[22] For example, a forty-year-old man, this would be 220 minus 40 (his age); his maximum heart rate would be 180 beats per minute during maximum physical exertion. This formula is applicable for both men and women. To obtain your heart rate after exercise press your finger on the carotid artery in your neck and count the number of beats for fifteen seconds; then multiply this number by four to obtain your heart rate for one minute. Your heart rate during physical exertion should not exceed your maximum heart rate.

3. **Target Heart Rate.** This is the desired range of your heart rate during aerobic activity. This range enables your heart and lungs to receive the most benefit from a workout without overexertion. This rate is contingent upon your physical condition, gender, and previous training experience. The intensity level should typically be in the range of 50 to 85 percent of your maximum heart rate.[23] For example, if your maximum heart rate were 180 beats per minute, as in the previous example, then your heart rate during aerobic activity should be in the range of 90 to 153 beats per minute (50 to 85 percent of 180).

One way to complete your workout within the target zone is to start at the lowest part of your target zone (50 percent) for the first few weeks. Gradually build up to the higher part of your target zone (75 percent). After six months or more of regular exercise, you may be able to exercise comfortably at 85 percent of your maximum heart rate. However, you don't have to exercise that hard to stay in shape. Working out within the 50 to 85 percent target zone is adequate.[24] When you are training, it is important to be aware of your limits regarding the level of intensity.

4. **Recovery Heart Rate.** This is your heart rate for a fixed period of time after ceasing a physical activity.

For example if a forty-year-old man increased his heart rate to 180 beats per minute during maximum physical exertion, and then stopped his workout, the time it took for his heart rate to return to his normal resting heart rate would be of interest. A healthy, fit person's heart rate will begin to drop more quickly, moving toward his or her normal resting heart rate within a shorter period of time than an unfit individual. The higher the level of fitness, the faster the heart rate will drop to a normal heart rate after intense exercise. Failure of your heart rate to drop quickly can be an indicator that you have overexerted yourself for your present fitness level. Challenging workouts are healthy, but the degree of challenge should be consistent with your fitness level. Failure to follow this principle may actually result in death.

Check your heart rate (as directed above) after you stop exercising. Then check it again after one minute, two minutes, and three minutes. If you are operating within your fitness level, your heart rate should become significantly lower after each minute.

Cholesterol

What is cholesterol? It is a soft, waxy substance found among the lipids (fats) in the bloodstream. It is an important part of a healthy body. Cholesterol is instrumental in the formation of cell membranes and certain hormones. Cholesterol is transported to the cells by special carriers called lipoproteins, but two kinds of cholesterol in particular are of interest:

- **HDL:** high-density lipoprotein (good cholesterol)
- **LDL:** low-density lipoprotein (bad cholesterol)

Cholesterol will not mix with water, so it needs assistance to travel throughout the blood stream. Packets of HDL cholesterol are formed to help move cholesterol through the blood, and approximately one-third to one-fourth of blood cholesterol is carried by HDL. HDL cholesterol transports cholesterol to the liver where it is excreted from the liver into bile—either directly or after conversion to bile salts. Excess cholesterol in your body can lead to the buildup of plaque in your artery walls. Plaque buildup can lead to narrowing, hardening, and blockage of the arteries.

The liver plays a central role in regulating cholesterol levels in the body. The liver synthesizes cholesterol for export to other cells and also removes cholesterol from the body by converting it to bile salts and excreting it into the bile. A high HDL level offers protection against heart attacks. A low HDL level indicates a greater risk of a heart attack and may also increase the risk of a stroke.

Low-density lipoprotein (LDL or bad cholesterol) is the major cholesterol carrier in the blood. If too much LDL cholesterol circulates in the blood, it can slowly build up in the walls of the arteries that feed the heart and the brain. With other substances, it can form plaque—a thick, hard deposit that can clog those arteries, causing a condition called atherosclerosis. A clot that forms near this plaque can block the blood flow to part of the heart muscle and cause a heart attack. If the clot blocks blood flow to part of the brain, a stroke occurs.

The real dangers of high cholesterol readings and ratios are that they increase risks for heart attack, heart disease, stroke, arteriosclerosis, coronary heart disease, and other cardiovascular diseases.

Cholesterol Guidelines

Measuring total cholesterol requires a blood test that indicates both LDL and HDL levels. The number is reported in milligrams per deciliter (mg/dl).

1. Ideal HDL (good) cholesterol: more than 40 mg/dl for men and more than 50 mg/dl for women.

2. Low HDL (good) cholesterol: less than 40 mg/dl for men and less than 50 mg/dl for women.
3. Ideal LDL (bad) cholesterol: less than 160 mg/dl.
4. Ideal LDL (bad) cholesterol for people with heart disease: less than 100 mg/dl, with 70 mg/dl being an ideal target.
5. High LDL (bad) cholesterol: 160 mg/dl and greater.
6. Ideal total cholesterol (HDL + LDL): less than 200 mg/dl.
7. Borderline high total cholesterol (HDL + LDL): 200–239 mg/dl.
8. High total cholesterol (HDL + LDL): 240 mg/dl and above.[25]

The most important number in predicting heart attack, heart disease, stroke, arteriosclerosis, coronary heart disease, and other cardiovascular diseases is the cholesterol ratio. You need to determine your HDL ratio. This ratio is computed by taking your total cholesterol and dividing it by your HDL number. If your total cholesterol is 240 and your HDL is 60, for example, divide 240 by 60; this would be an HDL ratio of 4.0. The chart below indicates your cardiac risk based upon your HDL ratio.

Cardiac Risks: (Cholesterol/HDL Levels)

Relative risk	Men (Ratio)	Women (Ratio)
Very Low	3.4	3.3
Low	4.0	3.8
Average	5.0	4.5
Moderate	9.5	7.0
High	>23	>11[26]

Reducing Total Cholesterol Levels

It is estimated that more than one hundred million American adults have elevated total blood cholesterol levels. There are a number of factors that can cause high cholesterol levels:

1. Diets with too much saturated fat (which raises LDL to higher levels)
2. Insufficient physical activity
3. Obesity or being overweight
4. Smoking
5. Stress
6. Advanced aging

The obvious ways to reduce cholesterol levels are to eat healthier foods, become more active, reduce excess weight, stop smoking, and practice stress management. Exercise is one of the best things you can do to develop your overall health and improve your cholesterol levels. Keep active and your LDL will decline while your HDL increases. Just what the doctor ordered! This can often be done without prescription drugs.

Eating a handful of nuts every day, especially walnuts, is a healthy habit to develop, as is eating three portions of fish each week—especially fatty fish like wild-caught salmon, mackerel, lake trout, sardines, and albacore tuna. Avoid eating lunch meats, high-fat dairy products, baked goods, fried foods, coconut oils, simple sugars, and syrup. These food products increase arterial inflammation, which promotes plaque buildup and increases LDL (bad) cholesterol in the bloodstream.

Vitamins taken in conjunction with a healthy diet can help control cholesterol. The following supplements are desirable:

1. A multivitamin that includes 1,000 to 1,200 International Units (IU) of vitamin D. Many trials and studies have linked low levels of vitamin D in the body to high levels of LDL (bad) cholesterol. Vitamin B has a proven

track record of lowering LDL cholesterol and raising HDL (good) cholesterol. This is especially true with niacin (vitamin B-3). Each of the B-complex vitamins has its own structure and performs its own function in your body. Note the recommended/optimal daily intake for the B-complex vitamins in the chart located in the appendix.

2. Six hundred milligrams of vitamin C (twice a day). Vitamin C promotes the presence of HDL, which reduces the more dangerous cholesterol (LDL) that causes so many problems.

3. Four hundred IU of vitamin E each day. Vitamin E assists by keeping LDL from going rancid and clogging arteries.

Prostate-Specific Antigen (PSA)

Prostate-specific antigen (PSA) is a protein produced by the cells of the prostate gland. PSA is present in small quantities in the serum of men with healthy prostates, but is often elevated in the presence of prostate cancer, which is the number one cause of cancer in men. The PSA level is checked through a blood test that assesses the amount of prostate-specific antigen present in the blood. It is considered the most effective test currently available for the early detection of prostate cancer. This is not a totally reliable test (since fifteen percent of prostate cancers occur in men with normal readings), but it serves well as a gauge.

The upper limit of normal is 4.0 nanograms per milliliter and levels between 4.0 and 10.0 indicate the possible presence of prostate cancer.[27] Readings are based upon age-adjusted values and by how fast these numbers increase from one year to the next. PSA levels that increased rapidly in the year before prostate cancer was diagnosed predict which tumors are deadly nearly ten times better than the PSA level itself. The change in PSA level from one year to the next is a more important health concern than the PSA reading itself. PSA numbers between 4.0 and 10.0 only serve as a gauge. It is recommended that men older than fifty have both a rectal exam and a PSA test annually. The best way to have any influence over the PSA number is by living a healthy lifestyle.[28]

Body Weight and Composition

Excess body weight is a risk factor for a number of debilitating diseases. For every additional pound of body weight that you carry, there are up to five more pounds of stress on the knee and hip joints.[29] Though joint replacement surgery is at an all-time high in America, most joint replacements last for only about ten years. Since one pound of excess body fat contains approximately one mile of capillary tubing, excessive body weight places more pressure on your body's effort to pump blood throughout your body. Prevention is the cure.

There are two other significant factors impacting body weight: muscle mass and bone density. Muscle mass is a significant factor in establishing an ideal weight, especially for body builders. Muscle is a healthy tissue, and a pound of muscle takes up less mass than a pound of fat. The presence of muscle is an excellent way to increase one's metabolism. Each pound of muscle burns between thirty-five and fifty calories each day, while each pound of fat on your body burns only two to four calories each day.[30]

Bone structure is a small factor in determining your ideal weight. Bones account for approximately 20 percent of body weight. When comparing two people who each weigh two hundred pounds but have extremely different bone structures, there is only a six-pound difference in the weight of their bones.[31] Resistance training is the best thing one can do to maintain bone density because it is a bone-stimulating activity that helps to prevent osteoporosis and decreases the aging rate of your heart, arteries and immune system.

There are many real and significant dangers of being overweight. Risk factors for health problems increase as your body weight exceeds a healthy figure. Among the physical risks are heart disease, heart attack, congestive heart failure, stroke, type 2 diabetes, metabolic syndrome, cancer, osteoarthritis, sleep apnea, abnormal blood fats (cholesterol), reproductive problems, gallstones, and joint stress (which may call for joint replacements).

The financial cost of medical care is high. The United States presently spends approximately 15.2 percent of our gross domestic product (GDP) on health costs.[32] This expenditure is expected to grow to 19.5 percent of our GDP by 2017. The cost is $2.3 trillion or $7,600 per person.[33] Preventive behaviors can do much to reduce this financial cost. It must also be noted that approximately 16 percent of people in the United States or forty-five million people have no form of health care.[34]

Being overweight is a preventable problem and can be controlled by making a few lifestyle changes. A healthy diet with portion control along with a balanced exercise program including body-resistance exercises, aerobics, and walking can eliminate excess body weight and the related health issues.

Body Mass Index (BMI)

The body mass index chart is a medically approved tool that assigns a number based upon your height in inches and your body weight in pounds. This number is used to evaluate whether or not you are within a normal body weight range for your height. It is the most widely used diagnostic tool to identify obesity within a population.

Body Mass Index Guidelines

Class	Body Mass Index
Severely underweight	Under 16.5
Underweight	16.5–18.4
Normal weight	18.5–24.9
Overweight	25.0–29.9
Obese	30.0–34.9
Clinically obese	35.0–39.9
Morbidly obese	40.0 and over[35]

Jim Williamson, BS, MA, EdS

Body Fat Percentage

Body fat percentage is a measure of the percentage of fat your body contains. For example, if you weigh 180 pounds and have 10 percent body fat, this means that you have 18 pounds of fat on your body and 162 pounds of lean body mass (bone, muscle, organ tissue, blood, and everything else). The amount of body fat makes a difference in your body shape and your overall health. Your goal should be to reduce excess body fat.

The following chart outlines the range of body fat percentages for the different levels of fitness.

Body Fat Percentage Guidelines

Classification	Women (Fat Percentage)	Men (Fat Percentage)
Essential Fat	10–13	2–5
Athletes	14–20	6–13
Fitness	21–24	14–17
Acceptable	25–31	18–24
Obese	32+	25+[36]

It should also be understood that a certain amount of fat is essential for bodily functions. Fat regulates body temperature, cushions and insulates organs and tissue, and is the body's main form of energy storage.

There are basically three ways to determine your body fat percentage:

1. **Bioelectrical Impedance.** This is when a very low electrical signal is sent through your body, usually accomplished by giving a person stand on sensors on a body fat monitor. The signal travels quickly through lean tissue, which has a high percentage of water and therefore is a good conductor of electricity. It travels more slowly through fat, which has a lower percentage

of water and is therefore a poor conductor of electricity. Bioelectrical impedance devices use the information from this signal to calculate your body fat percentage. This is a widely used method to *estimate* body composition. It should be noted that impedance measures may vary significantly because of differences in machines. In actual use, bioelectrical impedance analysis calculations of an individual's body fat may vary by as much as 10 percent of body weight. This variance makes it difficult for you to rely upon this kind of measure.

2. **Skinfold measurements.** This measure involves the use of a skinfold caliper to pinch predetermined areas on a person's body. The tongs pinch the skin, pulling the fat away from the muscles and bones. The gauge on the calipers measures the thickness of the pinch. It can be difficult to derive consistent measures using a skinfold caliper because the data is largely dependent upon one's ability to pinch the skin exactly the same way each time.

3. **Hydrostatic weighing tanks.** This method is both the most accurate and the most uncomfortable. A person sits on a scale in a large tank of water, blows as much of the air out of their lungs as possible, and then submerges in the water, staying underwater for five seconds while their underwater weight is recorded. The person being evaluated has to make sure that as little air is trapped in the lungs as possible, otherwise the test will be inaccurate, and the results will show a higher body fat percentage.[37]

Abdominal Size

People with an excessive abdominal size have the same health risk factors as people who have excessive overall body weight. Abdominal circumference measurements have proven to be useful in predicting disease. This measurement is taken at the level of the belly button. A male with a measurement greater than forty inches or a female with a measurement greater than thirty-five inches is generally considered to be at a high risk for disease.[38] The International Diabetes Foundation indicates that a waist measurement of thirty-seven inches for males and thirty-two inches for females are the upper limits of a healthy waist measurement.

Research has shown that abdominal fat may be more hazardous than fat in other areas of the body, but simply checking girth doesn't take proportion into account. That's why researchers considered height as well as waistline in establishing these numbers. The researchers found that men should have a waist-to-height ratio of 0.55 or less and women a ratio of 0.53 or less. To figure out what your maximum waist measurement should be for your height, take your height in inches and multiply it by 0.55 (for men) or 0.53 (for women). That will give you a good idea of the upper limit of a healthy waistline (in inches) for you. For example a man who is five-foot-ten should shoot for a waistline that is thirty-eight inches or less (70 x .55). For a woman who is five-foot-five, the upper limit for a healthy waistline would be thirty-four inches (65 x .53).[39]

Visceral or "deep" fat wraps around the inner organs and spells trouble for your health. How do you know if you have it? If you have a large waist or belly, you have visceral fat. Visceral fat increases your risk for diabetes, heart disease, stroke, and even dementia. Subcutaneous fat is found directly under the skin. It is the fat that is measured using skin-fold calipers to estimate your total body fat. This fat, in excess, is also considered to be a health risk if it is located on the belly.[40]

The health crisis can only be alleviated one person at a time. Increasing physical activity, developing healthy eating habits, and increasing your health knowledge are the foundation for better health. Newspapers, books, magazines, and the Internet are good sources for the information needed to make healthy changes, and much of the information that is available focuses on body weight. Why is body weight the predominant focus when people evaluate their health and the health of others? How much should you weigh? What guide should you use to evaluate whether you are too light or too heavy? What is the significance of your body weight when discussing your overall health? Is it just about physical appearance? Is there really such a thing as an ideal weight that contributes to the likelihood of having a healthy body? If so, what is the ideal weight for you?

Chapter 4:

So, I Want to Get Started - Now What?

We all know that there is a tremendous amount of health information available to us. With all of this information available, why is it so difficult for so many people to reach their ideal weight? Many of the obstacles that we face are mental. Our subconscious belief systems are the main culprit. For example, you may have a certain image regarding what your body should look like or a certain amount that you believe you should weigh. You may criticize yourself if you have not attained the standard that you believe you should. This mental process can leave you discouraged and feeling like you are not good enough. This can cause you to sabotage your efforts to attain a healthy weight.

Every time you make a decision to set a measurable goal and do not attain it, you may judge yourself too harshly. You may even see yourself as a victim. You may become sad or depressed. You may see yourself as a failure or a loser. This mental process is a definite hindrance to attaining a healthy body and an ideal weight. For many people, failure to attain the results they desire can have a lasting negative effect. When you give up hope because of past failures, it can be easy to stop trying. This is especially true if you attach some negative quality to yourself because of past failures. You may be plagued with thoughts of the past that affect how you think of yourself. They can cause you to think that since you failed in the past, you proved that you cannot do it—so, what's the use in trying again because you will likely fail? Chances for success are very unlikely when you think like this. Many times we fail only because we have approached a task with the wrong mind-set. Your mind-set when you approach any task or goal is very important to your success.

Instead of talking about losing weight, maybe it would be better to think in terms of gaining control of your weight. Maybe your focus should be on gaining more energy, setting a good example in helping your children to grow up healthier, or treating your body as though it was in fact the temple of the Holy Spirit. It is always better to focus on something that you are going to gain rather than on something that you are going to lose. Your mind tells you that when you lose something you want to find it again. This is exactly what happens with most diets, which have a 95 percent failure rate. When I began my lifestyle health program more than eight years ago, there were several things that I wanted to gain. I wanted a healthy blood pressure reading. I wanted to gain strength. I wanted to increase my endurance and gain freedom from medical visits. While I was focusing on what I wanted to gain, I happened to lose forty pounds with additional health benefits. To me, it always begins with *Why am I doing this? What am I trying to gain?* I recommend that you try this approach as you begin working toward your ideal weight.

Shifting Your Perspective

Understanding Your Motives

There are numerous reasons why people say that they want to reach their ideal weight. Remember that having a strong reason is a driving force that leads to success. What is your "why"? Without judging the appropriateness, some of the popular reasons include:

1. **Looking better.** For many people, personal appearance is a self-esteem issue. Often the purpose of wanting to improve one's appearance is to become more attractive

    to the opposite sex, to increase the odds of a new relationship, or to strengthen a present relationship.

2. **Improving personal health.** At a healthy weight, a person tends to feel better, have more energy, and reduce his or her risk of heart disease, stroke, diabetes, and high cholesterol.

3. **Shedding the stereotypes that are often attributed to those who are overweight.** Overweight people are often stereotyped as being stupid, lazy, unhealthy, unproductive, out of control, or unhappy. People who get out from under these stereotypes by losing weight often feel better both physically and mentally.

4. **Securing better employment.** You only have one time to make a positive first impression. There have been a number of studies that indicate that interviewers do, in fact, judge people by their appearance. Being overweight could very well result in not being hired for position that you are very qualified to fill. As mentioned above, overweight people are sometimes viewed as unproductive. If that is the perspective of an interviewer or potential employer, the overweight person is faced with a barrier to obtaining employment.

5. **Fitting into clothing.** Sometimes fitting back into clothing that you have outgrown symbolizes turning back the clock to your youth. It provides an opportunity to wear the clothes that you wore when you were younger. It can also be a financial issue. Changing sizes may require a greater outlay of money to replace clothing that no longer fits.

6. **Avoiding being made fun of.** Sometimes the cruelty and disappointment of being teased or ignored due to your weight can create a strong motivation to free yourself of those hurtful situations and your bruised feelings.

7. **Preparing for a special event.** There is evidence that some people are motivated to lose weight because of

upcoming events in their life. It may be a desire to lose weight because of a trip to a warm climate where less clothing is required. It could be because of an upcoming marriage, engagement, divorce, athletic competition, or class reunion. These types of events provide a special short-term motivation for some people to lose weight.

Most of these seven popular reasons for wanting to lose weight have little, if any, spiritual connection. The belief that your body is the temple of the Holy Spirit is the most spiritual reason for wanting to be a good steward of your body. Each person will ultimately determine their motivation for wanting to lose weight.

When you have accepted being overweight for a period of time and, as a result, develop a completely different mind-set toward your body weight, the decision to making healthy changes needs to be accompanied by a change in your mind-set that is tied to a reason why you want or need to change. It may be because of one of the reasons listed above, or it may be because of other reasons. Regardless of your reason, you should be aware of the medical risks of being overweight, and you should be making changes for the right reasons. Your desire to change should not be for someone else. It should be for you in hopes that you will gain something that you want. An acceptable motive to lose weight would be for the purpose of having a long and productive life. All changes begin first in your mind, and the change to reach an ideal body weight is no exception. When making changes, most people are motivated by what they want to gain from the change. Therefore, be clear regarding what you are hoping to gain from the change, and you will be off to a good start toward making those changes needed for your success!

Is it spiritually right to want to lose weight? Doesn't God love you unconditionally just the way you are? Is it worldly behavior to focus on wanting to lose weight? Are spiritual matters more important than physical ones?

Motives are expressions of the heart. It is possible to have wrong motives for just about everything. Let's consider a couple of wrong spiritual motives to lose weight. It is possible to desire to lose weight to provoke lust even when it masquerades as a desire to obtain good health. You may want to lose weight just for your personal pride. If the goal is to lose weight for the purpose of getting more attention as a result of a more attractive body, that is a pride issue.

Adopting a Lifestyle Change, Not a Diet

What you eat on a day-to-day, week-to-week basis is your diet. Therefore, everyone is on a unique diet. However, the term *diet* in America usually means a systematic way of eating and drinking designed to cause a person to lose weight. I located more than one hundred different types of diets that are advertised today.[1] That is a large number of specific types of diets. What is interesting is that even with more than one hundred different diets available, Americans continue to become more overweight and obese every year. It has been reported that people who diet to lose weight have a 95 percent failure rate.[2] You need to understand why diets in the past haven't worked. Diets are part of a multibillion-dollar industry. They tend to have little to do with changing people's eating habits. Anytime there is a focus on foods within a single food group or limited food groups, the diet is doomed for failure. Many diets are short-term plans with little hope of long-term success. You need a variety of foods for a balance of nutrients, and most diets are unbalanced. The following characteristics of the typical American diet may help explain why there is such a high failure rate:

1. People often approach diets with a certain level of dread. It is not often seen as a change to enhance the quality of one's life.
2. Diets are often seen as something people *need* to do, and they require us to deny ourselves the foods that we have come to enjoy. They are seen as unpleasant ventures in which we will need to give up things that we like for things that are not as desirable. That mind-set will present a problem at the very beginning of any diet.

3. Many people define a diet as a restrictive and painful process. It becomes more of an agreement to eat certain foods that they dislike but will eat in order to lose weight. This mind-set lacks promise for long-term success.

4. A diet is often seen as something you do to get weight off as quickly as possible, while all along thinking ahead to the day you can once again eat all of the foods that you are forced to avoid during the diet. This is another temporary mind-set.

5. A diet begins as a short-term solution to remove excess pounds that you desire to lose. This leads to the yo-yo syndrome of losing weight, gaining it back, and then starting the cycle all over again. This is very self-defeating.

All of these characteristics and observations doom the long-term success of a diet from the start. When a diet is dreadful or undesirable, you can expect little more than a short-term effect. If your main goal is just to attain a certain number on a scale, it is very unlikely that this goal will be compelling enough to sustain your effort for a long period of time. Even those who are able to attain that desired number on the scale tend to celebrate and then proceed to gain back the weight they lost.

Now contrast a *diet* with a *lifestyle change*. A lifestyle change requires a very different mind-set to lose weight. These are some characteristics that typically accompany a lifestyle change:

1. A lifestyle change is not perceived as dreadful, but is viewed with the anticipation of the positive benefits that are going to be realized in the future. There is a sense of eager expectation to achieve results: better health, the ability to be a better role model for others, and a consistency with Biblical principles.

2. A healthy lifestyle change is viewed as a way to provide proper nutrition and fuel to your body so that it will operate more efficiently. Failure to provide the proper

nutrition can create undesired illnesses and breakdowns that reduce the quality of your life. This was what I experienced, and it motivated me to make some lifestyle changes.

3. A lifestyle change is *not* for the short term. It is a change that is sustainable throughout your life. The end results should be so positive that the desire to go back to the old way is diminished in your mind. Maybe I was fortunate to have experienced poor health due to my unhealthy habits. Without that experience I might not have been motivated to change. Because of the positive benefits that I now experience, a healthy lifestyle makes sense to me.

4. Small lifestyle changes can result in significant positive results. Changes in the types of foods that we choose to consume have a cause-and-effect relationship. Healthy foods produce healthy results. You can begin to experience the positive effects of healthy lifestyle changes very quickly. This was my personal experience and the experience of others who have followed the Healthy Vessels program. For example, program members were able to discontinue different medications they were taking for their health. (These mediations had been prescribed to them before beginning the program.) In essence, you are what you eat: what you choose to feed your trillions of cells each day will dictate the health of your body.

5. Lifestyle changes are believed to serve as strong preventive measures in helping us avoid a number of serious health problems like heart disease, cancer, stroke, diabetes, arthritis, joint replacements, and many uncomfortable health irritations that impact our quality of life. Prevention of debilitating diseases is seen as a wise choice since the consequences of poor health are very expensive and may be impossible to reverse! Numerous

studies demonstrate this reality. Though there are no guarantees, does it make sense to take foolish risks?

I have tried various diets throughout my life and failed 95 percent of the time. When I engaged in periodic diets, I would lose weight, gain it back, lose it again, and eventually gain it back again. There was no long-term success because there was no long-term plan. Diets that focus only on helping you lose a certain amount of weight are only temporary plans. For the past eight years, I have adopted a lifestyle change, and there is no comparison regarding my energy and fitness levels. The ability to avoid medical problems was a reward in itself. I have a greater peace of mind and confidence about the lifestyle changes that I am presently implementing. My need for medical intervention has been eliminated, and my weight no longer fluctuates as it once did.

Setting Yourself Up for Success

Figuring Out Your Caloric Needs

With all of the conflicting health information that is available, it is helpful to have a basic knowledge of some dietary terms that are associated with weight gain and loss. For nutritional purposes, a calorie is a unit of energy-producing potential equal to the amount of heat that is contained in food and released upon oxidation by the body. On a practical basis, calories are units of energy.

Most foods and drinks contain calories; however, the number of calories varies greatly among food and drink choices. This makes it very important to become familiar with food labels in order to understand just how many and what type of calories a food or drink contains. By reading food labels, you can learn the number of grams of carbohydrates, proteins, and fats that are in a serving of food. Most food labels also designate the number of calories per serving. One of the best ways to become acquainted with nutritional information is by purchasing a calorie-counting book. The most useful books list the caloric content of many types of foods, and they state the number of grams of protein, carbohydrates, and fat in those foods.

The number of calories you consume over time will have a direct impact on how much you weigh. For every 3,500 calories that you consume beyond what your body requires, it will result in a gain of one pound. Calories are calories. To lose one pound of body weight, you must burn off 3,500 calories more than your body needs.[3] To lose that pound you can cut back on caloric intake to create a deficit or increase activity to burn more calories. Your best strategy for losing weight is to do both: reduce caloric intake and increase your activity level. Combining these two strategies will speed up the weight loss process and make it easier to maintain your desired body weight.

So, how do you maintain your present weight? In most cases you can maintain your present weight by limiting daily calories to between twelve and sixteen times your bodyweight. The number of calories that you need to obtain a healthy weight is not a number that is set in cement and applies to everyone at all times. Why? Your caloric needs will depend upon your current weight, metabolic rate, and activity level. You should record and monitor caloric intake for two weeks to determine the right number of calories to maintain your present weight. This step is necessary because there is quite a difference in calories consumed between twelve times your body weight and sixteen times your body weight. In our example above, twelve times two hundred pounds is 2,400 calories each day, but sixteen times two hundred pounds is 3,200 calories per day. As you can see, this is quite a range. At a similar caloric consumption, some people would maintain their weight; some would lose weight; and some would gain weight. Your metabolism and activity level will be the major factors as to the desired number of calories you must consume to maintain a particular body weight. Recording and monitoring your caloric intake over a period of time is the best way to determine the impact of caloric intake on your body weight.

When trying to lose weight, you should consume the number of calories that is equal to ten times your body weight, but never less than 1,200 calories per day or more than 2,000 calories per day. It will be difficult to maintain proper nutrition and to avoid losing muscle mass if you consume too few calories per day. When trying to lose weight, the goal is to lose unnecessary body fat, not muscle mass. When you take in too few calories, you will begin to lose both fat and muscle mass. That is neither healthy nor desirable. Taking in too few calories or taking in too many calories can be a problem. When you engage in a "starvation diet," your metabolism begins to slow down. Starvation mode decreases your metabolism, as a means to conserve energy and prevent starvation. Eating too few calories keeps your body from acquiring an adequate amount of nutrients and may cause you to *gain* weight in the long run. To acquire a long-term benefit, losing weight should always occur gradually without depriving your body of necessary nutrients. Depending on how much you weigh and how much you need to lose, it may be healthy to lose between two to four pounds each week. The first week of your lifestyle change often results in the most weight loss. That was my experience.

Regardless of the number of calories, it is imperative that consuming a balanced diet with proper nutrients becomes your focal point. You can lose weight and not be healthy. Your emphasis should not be just on losing pounds, but rather on promoting healthy eating and lifestyle changes. The goal of healthy eating is to nourish the trillions of cells in your body. If a healthy body is desired, calories need to come from nutritious foods. Excessive body weight is a health risk factor. Balance is the key! See the sample daily eating record in the appendix for an example of how to record your meals, calories, protein, carbohydrates, and fats. You can record your daily eating on one page in a notebook.

Recording may seem tiresome at first, but since most people tend to underestimate the amount of food that they eat, it is unlikely that you will have an accurate picture of your caloric intake unless you record what you eat each day. This is an effective way to organize and monitor your caloric intake. By documenting what you eat for a week at a time, you can observe the results of your eating changes. Did you gain weight? Did you lose weight? Did your weight remain the same? If your caloric intake is producing the results that you desire, you will want to continue until you reach your desired weight. If not, you will need to adjust your caloric intake and/or your activity level.

Monitoring Portion Sizes

An alternative way to monitor foods without keeping detailed caloric records is to monitor the portions of foods that you eat. I recommend that you eat five to six smaller meals each day. These meals should be approximately three hours apart. The key word in this strategy is *smaller* meals. These meals would include the following:

1. The first meal should consist of:
   a. one portion of a lean protein (A portion size is four ounces, approximately a size that would fit in the palm of your hand. Choices may include: chicken, beef, turkey, fish, beans, etc.);
   b. one portion (between one-half and one cup) of a healthy vegetable such as broccoli, Brussels sprouts, green beans, sweet potato, cauliflower, or some other low glycemic carbohydrate. Foods with a low glycemic index (55 or less) contain carbohydrates that break down slowly resulting in a gradual rise in your blood glucose levels. They also create a feeling of fullness for a longer period of time.
   c. one portion of another healthy carbohydrate *or* a healthy fat. You might eat an apple, banana, berries, unsalted nuts or other healthy choices (see the vitamins and minerals chapter). If the selection is fruit, it should be one whole fruit (apple, orange, banana, etc.). If it is something other than fruit, you should follow either the serving size listed on the food label or a portion size between one-half and one cup.

4. The second meal (snack) should take place three hours later. You would include a serving of a healthy carbohydrate or fat and a serving of a healthy protein.
5. The third meal should consist of the same amounts of food as the first meal above.
6. The fourth meal (snack) should be similar to the second meal/snack above.
7. The fifth meal should be like the first and third meals.
8. The sixth meal/snack should be like the second and fourth meals. If your caloric requirements (ten times your body weight; minimum 1,200 calories and maximum 2,000 calories) allow for more food, include this sixth meal. If not, you may choose to have only five smaller meals each day. Additional information is available on healthy proteins, carbohydrates, and fats in chapters 5 and 7.

The above information outlines the eating guidelines that you should follow as you are working to lose unhealthy weight. You should be eating five or six smaller meals each day that are within your caloric intake goals. You will initially find that it takes some added discipline to change your eating habits. Writing down what you eat is just one of the steps that you should take as you strive to be more disciplined about your eating.

Increasing Your Activity Level

Another important component in your program to lose weight is your activity level. In order for you to set up your exercise program, you should review chapter 8 "Do I Really Need to Exercise? (The Answer Is Yes)." The most efficient way to lose unwanted weight is a combination of healthy eating and exercise. I recommend three days per week of weight-resistance exercise and at least three days a week of aerobic exercise. For those who cannot do aerobic exercises, I recommend a daily walking program of thirty to sixty minutes each day. An increase in activity is needed to burn additional calories. The goal of increased activity is to require your body to break down your stored fat for energy.

Stored fat will not be utilized until your body needs it. When you create a situation in which you are burning more calories than your body is taking in, the fat reserves are called into action. This is the situation that you desire when your goal is to lose unnecessary body fat. If you are unable to begin with this schedule due to physical limitations, you should start within your physical capabilities. If you have questions as to what you can or should do at the beginning of your exercise program, you should contact your physician.

As previously discussed, for most individuals, the body mass index is an excellent gauge to predict ranges of desirable body weight. A normal body mass index reading is from 18.5 to 24.9. This figure should be used to determine whether your body weight is in the normal range. If your body weight is not in the normal range, the index can give you an idea of the target body weight that may represent your goal weight.

There are other factors to consider in determining a healthy body weight, such as body fat percentage and abdominal size (See chapter 3 "A Picture of Health"). When your body fat percentage and abdominal size are above healthy limits and your body mass index is higher than normal (above 24.9), it is fair to assume that you are overweight and that you would benefit from losing weight. It is likely that you are within healthy limits when your abdominal size and body fat percentage are in the healthy range even though your body mass index is slightly high. This situation is prevalent with bodybuilders and fitness practitioners. Because of their high percentages of muscle mass, their calculated BMI may fall into the overweight category on the chart. However, when considering how their weight is distributed, it should become obvious that they are not overweight. Abdominal measurement and body fat percentage are reliable indicators of fitness in these isolated cases.

Firing Up Your Metabolism

Increasing your metabolism is another way to help you drop unhealthy body weight. Metabolism is the rate at which your body burns calories.

Your metabolism slows down about 5 percent per decade after age forty. Much of this slowing has to do with the fact that your body tends to lose muscle mass as you age. The connection between muscle mass and metabolism is that people who have more muscle mass have a greater metabolism rate because more calories are needed to sustain muscles than other body tissues. Muscle burns more calories at rest than fat does; therefore, the more muscle mass you have, the faster your metabolism. It has been estimated that the average person loses approximately half a pound of muscle per year after age forty. Unless you take action, your metabolism will continue to slow down and make it easier for you to gain unwanted body weight. You can preserve muscle mass and slow the loss of muscle mass by engaging in strength-building activities. Men generally burn calories more quickly than women because they usually have more muscle tissue.

Some people believe that they cannot lose weight because their metabolisms are too slow. They may think that their metabolisms were locked-in at birth and cannot change. This is not true. It has been estimated that heredity is only about 5 percent responsible for a person's metabolic rate. Your metabolism can be increased and decreased by the lifestyle choices that you make. If your goal is to lose unhealthy weight, consider some of these practical ways to increase your metabolism:

1. **Eat five or six small meals per day.** Even though you consume the same number of calories that you would in three meals, distributing your daily calories into five or six smaller meals speeds up your metabolism. By contrast, increasing the length of time between meals causes your body to go into a starvation mode. This slows your metabolism as a means of conserving energy

and preventing starvation. Skipping meals slows your metabolism even further. To speed up your metabolism, you need to have smaller meals approximately every three hours. This prevents your body from going into starvation mode.

2. **Drink eight to ten eight-ounce glasses of water each day.** Water has zero calories, and your body actually burns additional calories heating up the cold water that you drink and bringing it to your body temperature. Water can also assist in creating a sense of fullness.

3. **Increase your muscle mass.** Fat burns fewer calories than muscle, even when you are just sitting or sleeping. Every muscle cell that you gain constantly burns calories for you. This is just one of the reasons why doing weight-resistance exercises each week is so important. People with smaller amounts of muscle and larger amounts of fat have much slower metabolic rates. Every pound of muscle on a person's body burns more calories at rest than a pound of fat burns.

4. **Exercise regularly.** Regular exercise not only burns additional calories while you are exercising, but continues to burn additional calories when the exercising has stopped. Exercise works in conjunction with a healthy caloric intake to reduce excess fat from your body. Raising your heart rate during aerobic exercises increases your metabolism. Exercise increases your need for energy; when coordinated with a healthy caloric intake, this energy must come from fat stored in your body. This utilization of fat speeds up the process of losing weight.

5. **Get adequate sleep.** Lack of sleep can decrease the number of calories your body burns just resting.

6. **Eat fish with omega-3 fatty acids.** EPA and DHA are the omega-3 fatty acids found only in fish oil. Fish oil increases levels of fat-burning enzymes and decreases levels of fat-storing enzymes in your body.

7. **Be more active.** When you are not doing a scheduled workout, find ways to keep moving. Never sit when you can stand, and never stand still when you can move. Movement in general helps to increase your metabolism by increasing your body's need for energy (burning more calories).

All of these factors work together in helping you to have a healthy body weight. Eating healthy, regulating calories through portion control, drinking adequate amounts of water each day, increasing muscle mass through weight-resistance exercises, doing aerobics, walking, becoming more active, and eating smaller, more frequent meals during the day all work together to help you attain your desired body weight. Incorporating these elements into your lifestyle is the healthy way to get the long-term results that you desire.

PART II:

PERUSING INFORMATION CENTRAL

Chapter 5:

Is All Food the Same?

Studying nutrition pertains to learning about food and how your body uses food as fuel for growth and daily activities. The nutrients needed for a healthy body come from different food sources, so you must strive to find a balance of foods in your diet.

The food pyramid guide is a visual tool intended to help people create a dietary plan that is rich in nutrients and low in saturated fats, cholesterol, and other substances that pose risks to good health. The United States Department of Agriculture issued a revised version of the pyramid called MyPyramid in 2005.[1] MyPyramid contains eight food groups and two other categories: activity and discretionary calories.

This pyramid groups types of foods into categories to encourage people to choose a selection of foods from each of the major food groups. The goal is to eat a variety of foods as part of a well-balanced diet that provides all the necessary nutrients. The individual food categories in the MyPyramid are:

1. grains;
2. vegetables
3. fruits
4. oils and fats
5. dairy; and
6. meats, beans, fish, and poultry.

MyPyramid emphasizes the importance of adopting a daily exercise plan as an essential part of a healthy nutritional plan. People are urged to get a minimum of thirty minutes of moderate to vigorous exercise every day. You can access more information at www.MyPyramid.gov.

Some of the biggest changes from the previous pyramid guide include:

- an emphasis on physical activity;
- food recommendations provided in cups, ounces and other measures that may be easier to understand. (The former guide used "serving size" as a measure.);
- up to twelve sets of recommendations provided rather than just one recommendation for all people (These twelve sets are based upon one's sex, age group, and activity level.); and
- personalized nutrition information.

Each of the six food groups in MyPyramid is intended to guide you toward getting the balance of nutrients necessary to support a healthy body. These nutrients are the chemical substances that you get in your daily food choices. The grains are divided into two subgroups: whole grains and refined grains. The whole-grain food choices address your need for nutrient-rich carbohydrates that contain the fiber needed in your daily diet. Refined grains have had many valuable nutrients removed as a result of their processing.

The vegetable group is organized into five subgroups based on nutrient content—dark green vegetables, orange vegetables, dry beans and peas, starchy vegetables, and other vegetables. This vegetable group provides a variety of nutrient-rich carbohydrates with fiber content. The fruit group includes fruits and 100 percent fruit juices. The fruit group contains nutrient-rich carbohydrate food choices.

The dairy group focuses on your need for calcium and is divided into four categories—milk, milk-based desserts, cheese, and yogurt.

The meat and beans group focuses upon your need for protein, fiber and healthy fats in your diet. This group is divided into six groups—meats, poultry, dry beans and peas, nuts and seeds, eggs, and fats.

The oils group in MyPyramid provides recommendations for oils that are high in monounsaturated fats or polyunsaturated fats that are low in saturated fats. The oils from plant sources do not contain any cholesterol. These fats are contrasted with solid fats that do contain cholesterol. Healthy fats provide your body with important nutrients and antioxidants for cellular repair of joints, organs, skin, and hair. Eating a balanced combination of these nutrient-rich foods adds up to a healthy diet.

Foods from these groups are necessary for building, repairing, and maintaining cells and body tissues, regulating the body processes, and providing energy. You must consume a certain amount of nutrients to survive. Your body needs food for three main purposes: obtaining energy, and growing and repairing worn-out tissue. It is important to eat a balanced diet in order to meet the basic nutritional requirements necessary for good health.

Certain food choices promote health benefits for your body, and other choices do little or nothing to support a healthy body. The nutrients discussed above are essential for maintaining life. When certain nutrients are missing from your diet, you can suffer unpleasant symptoms or even diseases from these deficiencies. For additional healthy food sources, see the list titled "Healthiest Foods to Consume" in the appendix.

There are three basic groups of nutrients: carbohydrates, fats, and proteins. They provide the primary source of fuel for your body. When they are broken down by your body, they provide usable energy. Each of these nutrients is different in chemical makeup and in what they contribute to building a healthy body.

Jim Williamson, BS, MA, EdS

Carbohydrates:
Your Body's Main Energy Source

Carbohydrates are your body's primary source of energy. The World Health Organization recommends that about 55 to 75 percent of your energy requirements should be met by your carbohydrate intake.

There are two main types of carbohydrates: simple and complex. Simple carbohydrates are made up of a single basic sugar. They provide the sweet taste in our food. On consumption, these sugars are directly absorbed into the blood as glucose. Simple carbohydrates provide energy but typically lack the vitamins, minerals, and fiber that are needed for a healthy body. Fruit sugar and table sugar are types of simple sugars. Complex carbohydrates are combinations of different types of sugars. These carbohydrates take a longer time to break down into their elementary form and require more time for digestion. Foods that contain complex carbohydrates do not spike blood sugar levels and are healthier for your body. So while they cause blood sugar to increase slightly, it doesn't spike quickly. Eating complex carbohydrates has many health benefits including:

- controlled blood sugar levels;
- weight loss;
- increased energy;
- improved memory;
- decreased risk of heart disease; and
- reduced cholesterol levels.

Since simple carbohydrates are broken down quickly, they provide instant energy and cause blood sugar levels to rise rapidly. Simple carbohydrates cause the body to counteract this great rush of blood sugar by pumping out too much insulin, which then brings blood sugar levels back down rapidly. When this rollercoaster effect happens on an everyday basis, there is an increase in the storage of fat in the liver and the cells of the body. If this fat is not burned or used up, serious health consequences may follow, such as:

- increased risk of type 2 diabetes;
- memory loss;
- low energy;
- hunger;
- weight gain;
- fatigue;
- mood swings;
- increased risk of a heart attack;
- increased risk of certain types of cancer;
- insulin resistance;
- metabolic syndrome; and
- diabetes.

Some people refer to simple carbohydrates as the "bad" carbohydrates and the complex carbohydrates as the "good" carbohydrates. But the issue is really one of balance. Approximately 65 percent of your daily calories should come from carbohydrates. Simple carbohydrates should make up only about 10 percent of your daily calorie intake, and complex carbohydrates should make up about 55 percent.[2]

Technically, fiber is a carbohydrate. Unlike other carbohydrates, fiber passes through the body with minimal changes. The benefit of fiber is that it keeps your digestive system running smoothly. There are two basic kinds of fiber: soluble and insoluble. Soluble fiber dissolves in water and soaks up fluid in your stomach and small intestine; fats and cholesterol are also absorbed and eliminated. Insoluble fiber cannot be dissolved in water and moves through your body, cleaning up substances that you have eaten that may be harmful. It also speeds up the time it takes for food to get from the entrance of your digestive track to the other. With enough fiber, you can cut that time in half. Many complex carbohydrates provide abundant sources of fiber. Beans, peas, whole grains, fruits, and vegetables are excellent sources for dietary fiber. Importantly, fiber plays a key role in helping your body fight disease. Both the American Heart Association and the National Cancer Institute recommend we increase our fiber intake to twenty-five grams per day. The average American eats about a third of this amount.

The glycemic index (GI) is a scale used to indicate how fast a particular food can raise your blood glucose (blood sugar) in your bloodstream after the food is ingested.[3] Foods are rated between 0 and 100. The higher the number is, the faster that food can raise your blood sugar. The low glycemic carbohydrates range is 55 or less; the medium glycemic range is from 56 to 69, and a high glycemic index is between 70 and 100.

Most, but not all, low glycemic carbohydrates are of higher nutritional value and help you feel full longer because they are absorbed by the body at a slower rate. It is best to eat foods that do not cause rapid rises in blood glucose levels. For example, broccoli is a low glycemic carbohydrate (10) while pretzels are a higher glycemic carbohydrate (83).[4] Americans consume far too many high glycemic carbohydrates that provide little or no healthy nutritional value. One healthy lifestyle change for you should be to reduce the amount of simple carbohydrates (high glycemic) in your diet and to include more complex carbohydrates (low glycemic).

There are, however, some high glycemic carbohydrates that do have nutritional value (contain vitamins and minerals) and should be included in a healthy diet. An example would be nutrient-rich fruits. Regardless of the glycemic index rating of fruits, nutrient-rich foods should not be compared to other high glycemic foods that lack nutritional value ("junk food"). There is a significant amount of information on the Internet, in books, and in magazines that quantify the amount of nutrients contained in foods.

Fats:
An Essential Part of Your Diet

The body uses fats as a source of energy. The chemical name for fats is triglycerides, and there are two forms: saturated and unsaturated. It matters a great deal what types of fats you include in your diet. There are four types of fats that are available in our food sources. The "good fats" (monounsaturated and polyunsaturated) lower disease risk, while the "bad fats" (saturated and trans) increase the risk of certain diseases. The key to a healthy diet is to substitute good fats for bad fats, and avoid trans fats. Some healthy guidelines for fats include:

- incorporating more omega-3 fats in your diet each day;
- adding lean meats and low-fat milk to your diet;
- removing trans fats from your diet; and
- choosing liquid plant oils for cooking and baking.

There is a great deal of misunderstanding when discussing the different types of fats we eat. To help clarify, consider the following information:

1. **Saturated fats.** These are generally solid at room temperature. Foods with saturated fats raise the level of cholesterol in your blood; excess cholesterol is known to cause harm by clinging to the walls of blood vessels and potentially inhibiting the flow of blood. The blockage of blood vessels can cause a heart attack or a stroke. High levels of saturated fats raise your risk of heart disease. They are found naturally in many foods, but the majority of saturated fats come from animal sources, including meat and dairy products. It is recommended that less than 10 percent of the fats in your diet are saturated fats.[5]

2. **Unsaturated fats.** Unsaturated fats are derived from vegetables and plants. Certain unsaturated fats are considered essential nutrients because they are not produced by the body. They can only be derived from your daily diet. These unsaturated fats serve many important functions in your body, including regulating blood pressure and helping to synthesize and repair vital cell parts. The two types of unsaturated fats are:

    a. **Monounsaturated fats.** These fats are typically liquid at room temperature but start to turn solid when chilled. When consumed in moderation, these fats can help reduce the bad cholesterol (LDL) levels in your blood and lower your risk of heart attack and stroke. They also help maintain body cells. They are typically high in vitamin E, an important antioxidant that works to support good health. Sources for monounsaturated fats include avocados, natural peanut butter, many nuts and seeds, olive oil, peanut oil, cottonseed oil, and avocado oil.

    b. **Polyunsaturated fats.** An advantage of these fats is that they can help reduce the cholesterol levels in your blood and reduce your risk of heart disease when consumed in moderation. Polyunsaturated fats are found in foods such as wild-caught salmon, almonds, walnuts, trout, herring, and corn, soybean, safflower and flaxseed oils. It is recommended that 20 to 35 percent of your daily calories come from fats. Most of these fat calories should come from monounsaturated and polyunsaturated fats.[6]

3. **Trans fats.** Unlike saturated and unsaturated fats, trans fats are created in an industrial process; hydrogen is added to liquid vegetable oils to make them more solid. Another name for trans fat is partially hydrogenated oil.[7] Companies use trans fats in their foods because they are easy to use, inexpensive to produce, and last a long time. Trans fats raise your bad cholesterol (LDL) levels and lower your good cholesterol (HDL) levels. Eating foods containing trans fats increases your risk of developing heart disease and stroke. It is also associated with a higher risk of developing type 2 diabetes. Trans fats are found in many foods, especially fried foods like French fries and doughnuts and in baked goods like pastries, pie crusts, biscuits, pizza dough, cookies, and crackers. The American Heart Association recommends

limiting trans fats to less than 1 percent of your daily calories or approximately two grams per day. Because of the serious health implications of consuming trans fats, some areas of our country have already banned their use in restaurants, and there is now greater nationwide awareness of this health risk. More and more, we see "No Trans Fats" labels on packaged foods.

There are certain fatty acids that are manufactured in your body and others that can only be obtained by the food that you eat. These fats are classified as:

a. **Essential fats.** These are fats that your body needs to maintain a healthy body. Your body does not produce these fats, so they must be attained through your diet. These are fats that are needed by every cell of your body. The two types of essential fats are omega-6 fatty acids and omega-3 fatty acids. The ideal intake ratio of omega-6 to omega-3 is between one to one and four to one. Most Americans maintain a ratio much higher than desired. Since most Americans eat far too many omega-6 fatty acids, the inclusion of more omega-3s will enhance a healthy ratio. This will help to combat inflammatory conditions and strengthen our immune systems. Consuming healthy amounts of omega-6 and omega-3 oils helps to lower high blood cholesterol and triglyceride levels, regulates diabetes by stabilizing insulin and blood sugar levels, and relieves water retention.

b. **Nonessential fats.** They are called nonessential because your body has the ability to produce them from fats in your foods. Nonessential fats include omega-9 (monounsaturated), omega-7, and saturated fats.

Jim Williamson, BS, MA, EdS

Proteins:
The Building Blocks of Life

Proteins, like carbohydrates and fats, are also compounds that contain carbon, oxygen, hydrogen, and nitrogen. The cells of the body are mainly composed of protein. Proteins are digested and used for the generation of new cells and the repair of damaged cells, including muscles, blood, skin, internal organs, hormones, and enzymes. Every one of the trillions of cells in your body is composed of proteins made from amino acids. A healthy body needs twenty-six amino acids. Proteins are made from amino acids, and both are referred to as the building blocks of life. Amino acids regulate every biochemical reaction in your body. They can exist singly or bound together, just a few or as many as five hundred in a chain.

Amino acids are used in every cell of your body, and they build the proteins you need to survive. Each one of the twenty-six amino acids is a little different. There are two classes of amino acids: essential and nonessential. Amino acids make up more than forty thousand proteins in your body. Since your body synthesizes seventeen amino acids naturally, it is essential that the remaining nine come from a healthy diet.[8]

Proteins that come from animal origin usually have all of the essential amino acids. Complete proteins are those that have all of the essential amino acids; incomplete proteins are missing one or more of the essential amino acids. Typical complete proteins include meat, fish, cheese, and milk. Incomplete proteins typically come from plants. Examples include wheat, corn, rice, and beans. When you consume too little protein, your body will use its own protein as a source of energy. However, there is not a lack of protein in the typical American diet. It is estimated that the average American consumes one and a half to two times the amount of protein needed for a healthy diet. Your protein needs depend on your age, size, and activity level. The standard method used by nutritionists to estimate your minimum daily protein requirement (in grams) is to multiply your body weight in pounds by 0.37.[9] According to this method, a person weighing 150 pounds should eat a minimum of fifty-five grams of protein per day, and a two-hundred-pound person should eat a minimum of seventy-four grams of protein per day.

If protein is taken as a supplement, the best delivery system is capsules rather than tablets. This is because the heat and pressure used to make most tablets can destroy amino acids. Protein supplementation makes it possible to obtain large amounts of protein with fewer calories and less fat than are usually obtained in high-protein foods. For instance, in one product used for supplementation, one scoop of whey protein can give your body approximately 120 calories, twenty-three grams of protein, three grams of carbohydrates, and two grams of fat. In comparison, four ounces of extra lean ground beef will provide 265 calories, twenty-one grams of protein, no carbohydrates, and nineteen grams of fat.

Water:
A Necessity for All Bodily Functions

In addition to carbohydrates, proteins, and fats, another important nutrient is water. Water plays a part of many necessary functions in your body and as a result is a key element in maintaining good health. Water makes up approximately 67 percent of the human body.[10] All of your cell and organ functions depend on water for efficient operation. Water maintains good muscle tone, assists in weight loss, aids in maintaining clear and healthy skin, assists in the digestion and absorption of food, transports oxygen and nutrients to the cells, and aids in metabolism. Water lubricates the body, forms the base for saliva, regulates body temperature, helps to alleviate constipation and rid your body of wastes efficiently, and allows for greater muscle mass and recovery from exercise.

Eight to ten eight-ounce glasses of water per day is recommended to maintain an adequate supply of water for your body, but there are a number of water sources besides tap water and bottled water. Some foods have high water content, including many fruits and vegetables. Mild dehydration symptoms are often (but not limited to): thirst, loss of appetite, dry skin, skin flushing, dark colored urine, dry mouth, fatigue, or chills. When you lose 5 percent of the total fluid in your body, the following effects of dehydration are normally experienced: increased heart rate, increased respiration, decreased sweating, decreased urination, increased body temperature, extreme fatigue, muscle cramps, headaches, and nausea. When the body reaches a 10 percent loss of fluids, emergency help is needed immediately. Anything above a 10 percent fluid loss is often fatal. Symptoms of severe dehydration include: muscle spasms, vomiting, racing pulse, shriveled skin, dim vision, painful urination, confusion, difficulty in breathing, seizures, loss of consciousness, and abdominal pain.[11] Going without any water at all in any form for just a few days could result in death.

Now that you know that all foods do not possess the same nutritional values, you can see why it is important to consume those foods that are most likely to optimize your personal health. Millions of dollars have been spent on advertising to influence your eating choices. You are bombarded daily with ads concerning your potential food choices. Many of these ads promote foods that are not healthy choices. If being healthy is your personal priority, one guiding fact that should assist you in making wise eating decisions is that your body is only as healthy as your cells. It is important for you to know what you can do to have healthy cells. You only grow old when your cells grow old. You become tired when your cells are polluted and undernourished. You become sick when your cells get sick. Everything about your body and your health depends on the condition of your cells. It is only logical that you should keep your cells clean, healthy, and well nourished in order to stay healthy, energetic, and vibrant for a long time. You need to have a basic understanding regarding those foods and environmental factors that contribute to healthy cells. This knowledge can then guide you toward healthy choices.

Chapter 6:

You're Only as Healthy as Your Cells

Cells are the building blocks of all living things. The human body is composed of more than one hundred trillion cells in skin, blood, and organs.[1] These cells provide structure for your body, take in nutrients from food, and convert those nutrients into energy. Cells are composed of many parts that are responsible for carrying out a variety of specialized functions. Since the cell is the source of your body's energy supply, the health of your cells will determine the level of your health. In essence, you can only be as healthy as your cells are. If you desire to have a healthy body, cellular nutrition is absolutely essential. When your cells are nourished properly, you will experience an abundance of natural energy, a resistance to degenerative diseases, and an overall higher level of fitness.

To nourish cells properly, a few factors come into play:

- getting the proper nutrients in the right amounts to your cells;
- having a cellular membrane that is able to assimilate these nutrients and allow these nutrients to pass through the cell membrane into the cell; and
- having cells that are healthy enough to properly utilize these nutrients.

Jim Williamson, BS, MA, EdS

How Cells Do Their Job

Cells provide energy through the mitochondria within the cell. As small as a cell is, each cell contains hundreds of mitochondria. Every one contains a very unique pattern of DNA, and their job is to facilitate cellular respiration, transforming oxygen and nutrients into energy and water. Each cell is surrounded by a special cell membrane that acts as the cell's security gatekeeper. The cell membrane decides what goes into the cell and what should be kept out. Assimilation is the delicate process in which nutrition passes through the cell membrane wall and into the cell. The old saying "You are what you eat" should really be "You are what your cells assimilate."

For optimum cellular nutrition assimilation, the cell membrane must be soft, healthy, and flexible. For this to happen, your body requires certain amino acids and specific "good" fats. This necessitates the consumption of high-quality protein and essential fatty acids, which should include omega-3 fish oil. Tuna, herring, halibut, trout, and salmon are high in protein and omega-3 fatty acids. You should avoid trans fats because they inhibit the delicate assimilation process. When you do not nourish your cells properly, you invite disease.

Keeping Cells Healthy

The cell is the basic unit of your body. Cells group together to form tissues, and tissues group together to form organs. Organs group together to form your body systems. This is the foundation for cellular health. You must have strong cells to support good health. It is not possible to have unhealthy cells and have a healthy body. To keep your cells healthy you need to:

1. Provide proper nutrition to your cells. This includes eating healthy, nutrient-rich food sources and high-quality nutritional supplements.
2. Provide proper cell exercise. When you exercise, blood circulation bathes your cells in nutrients that you received from your diet and washes away toxic waste products.

Exercise provides strength, endurance, flexibility, and mental alertness and is an excellent stress reliever.

3. Provide a clean environment. Healthy cells need ample water and clean air.

4. Provide adequate protection. When your cells are nourished with nutrient-rich foods, your immune system is strengthened. This is your protection from bacteria, viruses, and cell mutations.

5. Provide a healthy mental attitude. A positive attitude is an asset in maintaining healthy cells. Negative thoughts can compromise your immune system and intensify pain. Laughter may, in fact, be the best medicine, since happiness contributes to healthy cells.

While your focus is on maintaining healthy cells, you must understand that there are potentially serious health consequences when you allow your cells to become unhealthy.

Oxidative Stress and Free Radicals

One of the main health risks to your cells is a condition known as oxidative stress. To understand the danger of oxidative stress, you need to understand some structural features of an atom. To maintain a healthy body, you must sustain a degree of stability with the atoms in your body. When there is instability, negative conditions take place in your body. Your atoms are stable when the electrons in the outer shell of each atom exist in an even number or are paired. When there is an unpaired electron in the outer shell of the atom, an unstable condition is created. A free radical is an atom or group of atoms that has at least one unpaired electron in the outer shell.[2] Free radicals steal electrons from other atoms, and then the depleted atom becomes another unstable free radical. These cells are easily breakable, which causes your cells to perform erratically. Damage to your cells causes tissues to begin to degrade, and this allows disease to occur. For example, the actual cause of heart disease is damage done by free radicals to individual cells within the arteries. Free radicals are the major cause of aging and degenerative conditions.

Because of the potential damage to your body and the resulting diseases, your goal should be to neutralize the free radicals in your body. Failure to do so results in a chain reaction, causing a cascade of free radicals. One free radical can initiate tens of thousands of chain reactions and cause tremendous harm to your body. Free radical damage can destroy cell membranes, disrupt crucial processes in your body, reprogram DNA, and form mutant cells. Free radicals aren't always bad. When your body does not have an excess of free radicals, there are some benefits:

1. White blood cells use free radicals to destroy both bacteria and virus-infected cells. These free radicals prevent immediate death from infection.
2. With the help of free radicals, the enzymes of the liver detoxify harmful chemicals.

So, while some free radicals are good to have, problems arise when an excessive number of free radicals overwhelm your body's capacity to control them. This situation is known as oxidative stress. Medical research has shown conclusively that oxidative stress is the root cause of more than seventy degenerative diseases.[3] More than 180 large studies have been conducted on this issue, and each study shows the same results: people with the highest levels of antioxidants (which neutralize free radicals) in their bodies have a much lower risk of having heart disease, stroke, cancer, diabetes, arthritis, Alzheimer's, dementia, macular degeneration, lupus, multiple sclerosis, and other serious health ailments. Sometimes the studies showed the risk factor to be 200 to 300 percent lower.

Antioxidants work to neutralize free radicals. Remember, a free radical is an atom with an unpaired electron in its outer shell. Since an antioxidant is stable with a paired or unpaired electron in its outer shell, it can loan one of its electrons to the free radical and stabilize it. This creates stability for the atom so that it is no longer a free radical. This is the reason why antioxidants are extremely important in your diet. Antioxidants keep free radicals from wreaking havoc with your cells. It should be becoming clearer that you need to more than just add a nutrient or two to your diet; your body needs to combat oxidative stress by embracing lifestyle changes to keep your cells healthy.

Conditions Increasing Free Radicals

It has been estimated that each cell in your body may get ten thousand free radical "hits" each day.[4] There are a number of unhealthy habits and conditions that cause an increase of free radicals in your body. These include:

- Smoking and secondary smoke
- Medications
- Alcohol
- Prescription drugs
- Lack of clean air to breathe
- Radiation
- Food preservatives and additives
- Pollution: air, water, chemicals
- Computer monitors and televisions
- Nutrient deficiencies
- Tap water
- Sunburn
- Stress
- Use of microwaves
- Eating foods with trans fats and saturated fats
- Canned foods with lots of sodium
- White breads and pastas made with refined white flour
- Packaged high-calorie snack foods, like chips and cheese snacks
- Frozen food sticks and frozen dinners
- Boxed meal mixes
- Sugary breakfast cereals

- Processed meats: hot dogs, bologna, sausage, ham, and other packaged lunch meats

Many of these products, habits and conditions are commonplace in the American culture. Therefore, a starting place for reducing the number of free radicals would be to eliminate or minimize some of the foods or environmental influences that increase free radicals.

But what other defenses can you utilize to get excessive free radicals under control? Antioxidants! Antioxidants convert toxic free radicals into harmless elements. This is the only way to neutralize free radicals once they are formed.

Fighting Free Radicals: The Role of Antioxidants

A healthy relationship between free radicals and antioxidants is one of balance. An antioxidant donates one of its electrons to the unstable outer electron shell of a free radical. This ends the free radical's electron stealing, which had the potential to cause a chain reaction in your body. The antioxidants do not become free radicals because they are stable with either one or two electrons. Antioxidants are like scavengers, picking up unpaired electrons to prevent cell and tissue damage.

In addition to the antioxidant-rich foods that you eat, your body manufactures antioxidants that defend your body against excessive free radicals. There are several enzyme systems in your body that scavenge free radicals; however, you need additional help when your body is confronted with a large number of free radicals. The theory regarding free radicals is that, as you age, the oxidative damage that your body has sustained over the years takes its toll, causing the level of oxidative stress to increase. Studies show that the origin of many degenerative diseases may be linked to oxidative stress. Too often the body is confronted with more free radicals than it can handle. When this happens, the benefits of cellular nutrition become more important in reducing and controlling the free radical problem.

Antioxidants: The Right Type and Amount

The highest antioxidant foods typically come from fruit and vegetable sources. The American Cancer Society recommends that, in order to provide antioxidant protection for your body, you should eat a minimum of five to eight servings of fruits and/or vegetables each day. This is excellent advice. Foods that come from plants are your greatest weapon in providing enough antioxidants for your body. Oxygen radical absorbance capacity (ORAC) is a measure that quantifies the antioxidant power of the foods that you eat each day. The specific amount of antioxidants that is needed each day is unknown; however, it is known that only a small number of Americans are eating the quantities of ORAC-enriched foods that are recommended for a healthy body. A key issue is not only how many antioxidants you need but what the source of these antioxidants is.

ORAC Values

Is there any way to gauge the potency of an antioxidant? Oxygen Radical Absorbance Capacity (ORAC) is a method of measuring antioxidant capabilities in foods and measuring how many free radicals a specific food can absorb. (The values are usually based upon one hundred grams or three and a half ounces.) A food is considered to be rich in antioxidants when its ORAC value is 1,000 or more for one hundred grams. The higher the ORAC value is, the higher the antioxidant potential.[5]

Scientists with the United States Department of Agriculture have published a list of ORAC values for plant foods that are commonly consumed by Americans (fruits, vegetables, nuts, seeds, spices, grains, etc.). These ORAC values can be viewed at www.ars.usda.gov.

Some of the main antioxidants include vitamins A, C, and E. Some of the other antioxidants sources are: L-Carnosine, carotenoids, co-enzyme Q-10, green tea, vitamin B, flavonoids, selenium, soy and isoflavones (found in soy beans), and zinc.

United States Department of Agriculture researchers believe that to provide meaningful antioxidant health benefits, you need foods that total a minimum of 3,500 to 4,500 in ORAC value in your daily diet. There is reason to believe that this recommendation is going to be increased. Recent studies indicate that the average human consumes less than 1,000 ORAC each day. A deficiency may lead to degenerative illnesses such as cancer, arthritis, or memory loss. These diseases have increased considerably in recent decades. In 2010, the expected incidence of cancer in the United States is 1.5 million compared to the 1.2 million cases in the year 2000. In 2003 arthritis affected approximately 43 million adults compared to an estimated 49.9 million adults in 2009. In the year 2000, 4.5 million Americans were diagnosed with Alzheimer's disease. This number has grown to 5.3 million Americans, and 454,000 new cases are expected to be diagnosed this year.

So what is the best approach to prevent or control oxidative stress? The best approach is to strengthen your body's natural defense through cellular nutrition. According to medical literature, one way to define cellular nutrition is "the providing of all nutrients to the cell at optimal levels that has shown to provide a benefit to your health." It is providing the body with all the antioxidants along with the supporting B vitamins and antioxidant minerals at optimal levels. This is preventive medicine at its best.

Free radicals are produced continuously in the human body. They are the by-products of your natural metabolic processes as you consume oxygen to create energy. All processes involving oxygen, including cellular respiration, cause the formation of free radicals. An excess accumulation of free radicals can damage cells and inactivate your cellular respiration. This can lead to the death of the cell. Your body's defense is to utilize antioxidant molecules to fight off the free radicals. Your diet will determine the antioxidant strength that you have to combat an excess of free radicals.

Supplementing Your Diet

Standards for the recommended daily allowances (RDAs) were developed in the 1920s to provide guidelines to avoid acute-deficiency diseases such as scurvy (vitamin C deficiency) and rickets (vitamin D deficiency). Since the RDA levels were originally determined for that purpose, they only apply to the minimum levels of nutrients needed to ward off those certain acute deficiency diseases, which are no longer common. This standard has little practical value today. Recent research indicates that to combat oxidative stress, it is necessary to provide your body with optimal levels of nutrients.

The optimal daily intake better represents what is required for proper cellular nutrition because the levels recommended are much higher than those proposed by the recommended daily allowances. For example, the optimal level of vitamin E is 400 International Units (IU). The RDA recommends only 10 to 30 IU. To ingest 400 IU of vitamin E, you would have to eat thirty-three heads of spinach, twenty-seven pounds of butter, eighty avocados, or five pounds of wheat germ every day. To consume enough food to meet the recommendations of the optimal daily intake of vitamin C, you would have to eat eighteen oranges or 160 apples. These choices are not very practical. Thus, for many people, some supplementation is desirable. The supplementation that you will need to take will have much to do with what nutrients you are getting or not getting from your diet. There is no one set of supplementation recommendations that can fit everyone. Supplementation decisions will differ depending upon your age, sex, daily diet, and activity level.

So, how can we obtain the optimal level of nutrients? The answer is twofold. First, you need to eat healthy foods, and second, you need to consume high-quality nutritional health supplements to boost your cellular nutrition to optimum levels. You need to focus on including the most potent antioxidants into your diet. Healthy eating would include consuming five to eight servings of fresh fruits and/or vegetables each and every day. In addition to eating fresh fruits and vegetables, you need to include high-quality supplements that support optimum cellular nutrition. One of the best supplement recommendations is to take fish oil (containing omega-3 fatty acids) capsules each day. Follow the recommendations on the label. Think of taking supplements as a form of preventive medicine to stop disease processes before they even begin. The goal is to get oxidative stress under control and keep it under control. It takes a minimum of six months to build up your body's natural defenses. For this reason, it is important that you follow healthy nutritional recommendations so that your body can build up its own defenses against disease. Having a strong immune system is critical in protecting your body from unwanted disease.

The concept of cellular nutrition today is very different from the approach that nutritional medicine focused on during the past fifty years. For many years, nutritional medicine narrowed its focus to ways to replenish nutritional deficiencies. Members of the nutritional medicine community invested most of their time and energy administering a large number of different tests to determine which specific nutrients people needed to supplement. For instance, if they determined that you did not have enough vitamin E in your diet, then the solution would be to add more vitamin E into your diet. In this approach, they were looking for the isolated culprit that was the cause of a nutritional problem. The main problem with this approach to nutrition is that vitamins are not drugs. They are natural nutrients that your body should get from the foods you eat. The various antioxidants and supporting nutrients work on different parts of your body. For example:

- Vitamin E is the best antioxidant within the cell membrane.[6]
- Vitamin C is most effective within the plasma.[7]
- Glutathione works most efficiently within the cell itself.[8]

Literally dozens of antioxidants are at work in various parts of your body and are effective against particular types of free radicals. Antioxidants work together, not in isolation, to control oxidative stress. It is difficult to understand this relationship when medical research separates these nutrients and tries to study the individual effect of each vitamin and mineral despite the fact that vitamins and minerals, in fact, work collectively.

What are some practical nutritional habits that will provide assistance in the battle with free radicals to reduce oxidative stress and promote optimal cellular nutrition? Consider the following:

- Eat a minimum of five to eight servings of fruits and/or vegetables each day.
- Take antioxidant supplements.
- Include a variety of antioxidants in your diet.
- Make sure that foods in your daily diet include a minimum ORAC value of 3,500 to 4,500.

Due to the importance of supporting healthy cells, it is important that you choose foods that contain the necessary nutrients. To gain a greater understanding of the nutrients in food, you will need to have a working knowledge of the vitamins and minerals that exist in food. This information will help you make informed food decisions. Healthy food choices and appropriate vitamin and mineral supplementation work hand in hand to promote healthy bodies.

Chapter 7:

Building Blocks for Life:
Vitamins and Minerals

I am convinced that the role of vitamins and minerals is one of the most confusing topics for many people. Though many people have a basic concept of what vitamins and minerals are, there is a knowledge gap when evaluating what vitamins and minerals are needed, in what quantities, in what forms, and from what sources. To further complicate matters, media sources offer conflicting information. One day a certain vitamin is mentioned as an absolute necessity; then another article will issue a warning that the same vitamin may be dangerous if the dosage is too high. You are told that certain vitamins and minerals are necessary to reduce the risk of developing certain health conditions, but this may be followed by another report that says there is no impact at all.

Trying to evaluate what you really need in your daily diet becomes confusing with all this contradicting information. First you are told the amounts of different nutrients that you need and then you hear terms such as milligrams, micrograms, and International Units. All this information leaves many people confused as to how these nutrients should fit into their daily eating habits. It is easier to eat those foods that are highly advertised and readily available than to try to figure out the nutritional value of foods for yourself.

Unfortunately, this is what is happening for millions of people, and this strategy is not necessarily in the best interests of your health.

My goal is to simplify the most current and generally accepted information into understandable terms. I will discuss the vitamins and minerals that are recommended for a healthy diet, explain their value, and identify the food sources in which they are found. This chapter will give you a basic understanding regarding the benefits of the recommended vitamins and minerals. It is important, however, to understand that vitamins and minerals work in concert with one another—not in isolation. My hope is that this will alleviate some of the confusion that exists regarding vitamins and minerals.

Vitamins

Vitamins and minerals are also called micronutrients. Though they do not contain calories to provide energy for your body, they are responsible for regulating all of your body functions. (For example, you need Vitamin A in order to see.) Vitamins are organic chemical compounds that are required for normal growth and metabolism. There are a total of thirteen vitamins that are divided into two classes: fat-soluble vitamins and water-soluble vitamins. There are four fat-soluble vitamins (vitamins A, D, E, and K) and nine water-soluble vitamins (the eight B vitamins and vitamin C). These two classes of vitamins have different qualities. Cooking and heating destroy the water-soluble vitamins more readily than the fat-soluble vitamins. Fat-soluble vitamins move through the body more slowly than the water-soluble vitamins, allowing for the possibility of an excessive toxic buildup. On the other hand, because water-soluble vitamins move through the body more quickly, they are more likely to be depleted quickly, resulting in a deficiency. Vitamin deficiencies can occur from an unbalanced diet, disease, drug interactions, and the consumption of medicines and antibiotics.

Vitamins are organic substances that are necessary for normal health and growth in both animals and humans. With the exception of Vitamin D, your body does not produce vitamins, so you must get them from your diet. It is best to get vitamins through a variety of healthy foods, but you may also get vitamins through dietary supplements. While vitamins prevent and cure some specific diseases, they are also necessary for virtually every function within your body.

Vitamins assist the enzymes that release energy from carbohydrates, proteins, and fats. Vitamins strengthen your immune system, support normal growth and development, and help your cells and organs do their jobs. When a vitamin is absent from your diet, or your body doesn't properly absorb it, a specific deficiency disease may develop.

A vitamin deficiency occurs when your body does not have enough of a particular vitamin to operate efficiently. Many people take vitamin and mineral supplements as a backup plan to ensure that their bodies are getting all the necessary nutrients. This is a good strategy.

As previously discussed, vitamins are either water-soluble or fat-soluble. We'll begin with a discussion of the nine water-soluble vitamins, the vitamin B-complex (8) and vitamin C. The eight B-complex vitamins are vitamin B1 (thiamine), vitamin B2 (riboflavin), vitamin B3 (niacin), vitamin B5 (pantothenic acid), vitamin B6 (pyridoxine), vitamin B8 (biotin), vitamin B9 (folic acid), and vitamin B12 (cobalamin). When water-soluble vitamins are taken, your body uses what it needs, and the remaining amount is discharged in urine. Water-soluble vitamins cannot be stored in your body, so you need to include these vitamins in your diet on a regular basis to assure that they are properly replenished. Water-soluble vitamins are easily washed away and even destroyed during regular food preparation. Cooking time, temperature, and cooking method are all factors that determine vitamin loss during food preparation.

Water-Soluble Vitamins

As the name implies, vitamin B complex is a combination of eight essential vitamins. Although each is chemically distinct, the B vitamins have common dietetic sources such as whole grains, legumes, eggs, dairy products, meat, and fish. They often work together to bolster metabolism, maintain healthy skin and muscle tone, and enhance the function of your immune and nervous systems. They promote cell growth and division, including that of the red blood cells that help prevent anemia. Together they also combat stress, depression, and cardiovascular disease. These vitamins are in charge of carrying out physical and chemical processes that keep you alive and healthy. An important thing to remember about the B vitamins is that they should be taken together. They are so interdependent in function that large doses of any of them may cause a deficiency in others. If you are not already taking a multivitamin and mineral supplement that contains the B vitamin complex, it may be helpful to add a B complex supplement. Included below are details regarding the recommended sources and health benefits of the water-soluble vitamins (B complex and C).

1. **Vitamin B-1 (thiamine).** B-1 is needed to process carbohydrates, proteins, and fats. Every cell of your body requires B-1 to form the fuel that your body runs on, called ATP. B-1 supports proper heart function, maintains your energy supplies, and coordinates the activities of your nerves and muscles. Nerve cells require Vitamin B-1 to function normally. B-1 helps fuel your body by converting blood sugar into energy, and it keeps your mucous membranes healthy. It is also essential for the nervous system and for cardiovascular and muscular function.

   Recommended food sources: asparagus, sunflower seeds, romaine lettuce, mushrooms, spinach, Brussels sprouts, tuna, green beans, tomatoes, pinto beans, Lima beans, navy beans, yellow corn, black beans, green peas, whole-grain cereals, rye, whole-wheat flour, wheat germ, and kidney beans.

Signs of shortage include: loss of appetite; "pins and needles" sensations; numbness, especially in the legs; muscle tenderness, especially in the calf muscles.

2. **Vitamin B-2 (riboflavin).** B-2 is needed to process amino acids and fats, activate Vitamin B-6 and B-9, and help convert carbohydrates into ATP, the fuel that your body runs on. In some conditions it can act as an antioxidant. It helps protect cells from oxygen damage. Your body needs vitamin B-2 for growth and red cell production. It also promotes healthy skin and good vision.

Recommended food sources: calf liver, venison, low-fat yogurt, soybeans, spinach, low-fat (2 percent) cow's milk, lean beef tenderloin, red meats, green leafy vegetables, dairy products, riboflavin-enriched breads and cereals, mushrooms, goat's milk, asparagus, romaine lettuce, steamed broccoli, boiled eggs, mustard greens, green beans, celery, cabbage, strawberries, raspberries, Brussels sprouts, and almonds.

Signs of shortage include: sensitivity to light; tearing of the eyes, burning and itching in and around the eyes; soreness around the lips, mouth, and tongue; cracking of the skin at the corners of the mouth; peeling of the skin, particularly around the nose.

3. **Vitamin B-3 (niacin).** The body uses B-3 in the process of releasing energy from carbohydrates. B-3 is needed to form fat from carbohydrates. It is important for converting calories from carbohydrates, proteins, and fats. It also helps your digestive system function; in addition, it promotes a normal appetite and healthy skin, and helps maintain the normal functioning of your nervous system. B-3 stabilizes your blood sugar

level; it helps your body process fats, supports the genetic processes in your cells, and helps lower your cholesterol levels.

Recommended food sources: baked or broiled tuna, roasted chicken breast, baked or broiled halibut, baked or broiled salmon, asparagus, milk, eggs, yeast, romaine lettuce, roasted turkey breast, tomatoes, mustard greens, green beans, baked or broiled cod, steamed broccoli, raw carrots, spinach, peanuts, raspberries, cantaloupe, boiled cauliflower, and lean beef tenderloin.

Signs of shortage include: generalized weakness or muscular weakness, lack of appetite, skin infections, and digestive problems.

4. **Vitamin B-5 (pantothenic acid).** B-5 is involved in the cycle of energy production. B-5 is essential in producing, transporting, and releasing energy from fats. Synthesis of cholesterol depends on B-5. This vitamin activates your adrenal glands, and a byproduct of B-5 is believed to lower blood levels of cholesterol and triglycerides. B-5 turns carbohydrates and fats into usable energy, improves your body's ability to respond to stress by supporting your adrenal glands, and assures production of healthy fats in your cells.

Recommended food sources: cauliflower, most beans (not green beans), lean meat, poultry, fish, whole-grain cereals, steamed broccoli, cooked turnip greens, sunflower seeds, tomatoes, strawberries, grapefruit, low-fat yogurt, boiled eggs, winter squash, collard greens, and yellow corn.

Signs of shortage include: fatigue, listlessness, sensations of weakness, numbness, tingling, and burning or shooting pain in the feet.

5. **Vitamin B-6 (pyridoxine).** B-6 is essential for processing amino acids, which are the building blocks of all proteins and some hormones. This vitamin helps convert protein to energy, and it is an essential nutrient in the regulation of mental processes and, possibly, mood. It works with folic acid and vitamin B-12 to reduce blood levels of homocysteine (an amino acid linked to heart attack, stroke, and possibly diseases such as osteoporosis and Alzheimer's disease). B-6 supports a wide range of activities in your nervous system and promotes the proper breakdown of sugars and starches.

   Recommended food sources: spinach, turnip greens, garlic, poultry, eggs, soybeans, oats, whole grains, cereals, nuts, seeds, fish, baked or broiled tuna, cauliflower, bananas, celery, boiled asparagus, steamed broccoli, kale, collard greens, Brussels sprouts, watermelon, cod, tomatoes, snapper, carrots, eggplant, cantaloupe, romaine lettuce, baked potato with skin, raw onions, chicken breast, sweet potato with skin, turkey breast, venison, lean beef tenderloin, baked or broiled salmon, flaxseeds, strawberries, pineapple, grapes, and avocados.

   Signs of shortage include: fatigue, anemia, convulsions or seizures, and skin disorders such as eczema and dermatitis.

6. **Vitamin B-7 (biotin).** B-7 acts as a coenzyme in the metabolism of protein, carbohydrates, and fats. This vitamin works to alleviate muscle pain and control muscle cramps; it also assists in the synthesis of fatty

acids and helps in energy metabolism and in the synthesis of amino acids and glucose.

Recommended food sources: milk, liver, egg yolk, legumes, nuts, meat, poultry, whole grains, soybeans, saltwater fish, romaine lettuce, carrots, almonds, eggs, cabbage, cucumber, cauliflower, raspberries, strawberries, oats, walnuts, onions, halibut, cow's milk, liver, salmon, carrots, bananas, yeast, cereals, and goat's milk.

Signs of shortage include: fatigue, skin rashes, loss of appetite, nausea, depression, muscle pain, hair loss, and lethargy.

7. **Vitamin B-9 (folic acid).** B-9 is needed for cell replication and growth. It is also needed to make normal red blood cells and to prevent anemia. B-9 helps to form the building blocks of DNA, the body's genetic information, and helps the building blocks of RNA, which is needed for protein synthesis in all your cells. Rapidly growing cells, such as those of a fetus, and rapidly generating cells, like red blood cells and immune cells, have a high need for folic acid (B-9). A diet low in B-9 has been associated with a high incidence of precancerous polyps in the colon.

Recommended food sources: green vegetables such as broccoli and asparagus, fruits, dried beans, nuts, mushrooms, fortified cereals, grain products, peas, liver, and cauliflower.

Signs of shortage include: fatigue, acne, sore tongue, cracking at the corners of the mouth, diarrhea, appetite loss, weakness, shortness of breath, headaches, irritability, heart palpitations, and depression. A severe deficiency can result in anemia and can slow the growth rate of children, and newborns are at risk of being born with spina bifida and other serious defects of the nervous system.

8. **Vitamin B-12 (cobalamin).** B-12 is needed for normal nerve cell activity, DNA replication, and production of the mood-affecting substance SAMe. B-12 keeps your nervous system healthy and acts with other B-complex vitamins to control homocysteine levels. It works with folic acid to produce healthy red blood cells. It is needed to make DNA.

   Recommended food sources: calf liver, baked or broiled salmon, venison, cheese, chicken, lean beef tenderloin, baked or broiled cod, baked or broiled halibut, low-fat yogurt, boiled eggs, and cow's milk.

   Signs of shortage include: red or sore tongue, tingling or numbness in feet, nervousness, heart palpitations, depression, memory problems, dandruff, decreased reflexes, difficulty swallowing, fatigue, nervousness, paleness, and weak pulse.

9. **Vitamin C.** This vitamin acts as an antioxidant that protects LDL cholesterol from oxidative stress. Vitamin C may protect against heart disease by reducing the stiffness of arteries and the tendency of platelets to clump together. Vitamin C is needed to make collagen, the "glue" that strengthens many parts of your body. It plays a role in wound healing as a natural antihistamine. It aids in the formation of liver bile and helps to fight viruses and detoxify alcohol and other substances. It improves the nitric oxide activity that is needed for the dilation of blood vessels; this is important in lowering blood pressure and preventing spasms in the arteries of the heart that might otherwise lead to a heart attack. It

may lower the risk of cataracts. It may protect the body from retaining or accumulating lead, a toxic mineral. It is instrumental in allowing your body to resist infection. Vitamin C helps to protect your cells from free radical damage, aids in the absorption of iron from food so that your body can fight anemia, absorbs calcium to assist in the formation of bones and teeth, supports a healthy level of blood sugar, lowers cancer risk, regenerates the body's vitamin E supplies, and lowers the risk of asthma.

Recommended food sources: bell peppers, steamed broccoli, cauliflower, strawberries, lemon juice, romaine lettuce, mustard greens, Brussels sprouts, papaya, grapefruit, kiwi fruit, turnip greens, cantaloupe, oranges, cabbage, tomatoes, raspberries, asparagus, celery, spinach, pineapple, watermelon, green beans, cranberries, blueberries, squash, carrots, garlic, apricots, sweet potato with skin, bananas, apples, beets, onions, pears, grapes, yellow corn, and avocados.

Signs of shortage include: poor wound healing, frequent colds or infections, lung-related problems, scurvy, loosened teeth, bruises, nosebleeds, and swollen, painful joints.

Fat-Soluble Vitamins

The four fat-soluble vitamins (A, D, E, and K) are organic compounds that are needed by your body in trace amounts. Like water-soluble vitamins, fat-soluble vitamins are essential to your health. Since we have an ample food supply in the United States, you should be able to obtain adequate amounts of fat-soluble vitamins in your diet without relying on supplements. Fat-soluble vitamins do not need to be replenished as often as water-soluble vitamins because they can be stored in the liver or in the fat tissues of your body until your body needs them—even up to six months.[1] When these stored vitamins are needed, special carriers in your body transport them where they will be utilized.

Fat-soluble vitamins are essential for protection against certain diseases. These vitamins can be found in both plant and animal sources. It is possible to have too much of a fat-soluble vitamin, and an excessive amount of a fat-soluble vitamin can result in a dangerous toxic condition. For this reason, it is unlikely that these vitamins will need to be supplemented as often as water-soluble vitamins. Listed below are the health benefits and recommended food sources of the fat-soluble vitamins.

1. **Vitamin A.** This vitamin plays a vital role in bone growth, reproduction, and the health of our immune systems. It helps skin and mucous membranes repel bacteria and viruses, and it acts as an antioxidant that helps protect your cells against cancer and other debilitating diseases, improves your vision, and helps prevent night blindness. It may slow down declining retinal function in some people. It helps prevent certain skin conditions, works against heart disease and stroke, aids in lowering blood cholesterol, guards against many types of infections, helps reduce wrinkles, helps eyes adjust to light changes, neutralizes free radicals that cause tissue and cellular damage, and helps fight diseases caused by viruses.

   Recommended food sources: raw carrots, boiled spinach, bell peppers, mustard greens, romaine lettuce, sweet potato with skin, collard greens, cantaloupe, apricots, steamed broccoli, tomatoes, boiled asparagus, squash, spinach, turnip greens, raspberries, boiled Brussels sprouts, cucumbers, watermelon, grapefruit, celery, prunes, papaya, green beans, cabbage, plums, oranges, and low-fat (2 percent) cow's milk.

Signs of shortage include: frequent viral infections, night blindness, the appearance of goose-bumps on the skin, and reduced ability to fight infections.

2. **Vitamin D.** This nutrient assures that children will have healthy teeth and bone development. It helps with any function that utilizes calcium or phosphorus, such as nerve transmission, the beating of the heart, and blood clotting. Vitamin D fights respiratory infections, aids in preserving bone mass, prevents diseases like rickets, helps regulate bodily functions, and assists in nutrient absorption. It helps prevent type 2 diabetes, multiple sclerosis, hypertension, osteoporosis, and certain cancers (including colon, prostate, breast, and ovarian). It regulates the growth and activity of your cells and reduces inflammation. Insufficient quantities of vitamin D lead to cell energy starvation, fatigue, headaches, muscle cramps, and allergies.

   Recommended food sources: Baked and broiled salmon, mackerel, tuna, margarine, liver, cheese, low-fat (2 percent) cow's milk, baked and broiled cod, cod liver oil, boiled eggs, sardines, herring, fortified orange juice, and mushrooms.

   Signs of shortage include: Bone pain and/or soft bones, frequent bone fractures, bone deformities, or growth retardation in children.

3. **Vitamin E.** This antioxidant protects your cell membranes and other fat-soluble parts of your body from damage that can occur due to the presence of LDL (bad) cholesterol. Vitamin E plays a role in your body's ability to process glucose and has a direct effect on inflammation, blood cell regulation, connective tissue growth, and genetic control of cell division. It can

prevent blood cells from sticking together, which helps promote clear and flexible blood vessels. It can protect your skin from ultraviolet light, prevent cell damage from free radicals, decrease the risk of coronary artery disease, aid in proper blood clotting, aid in healing of wounds, and help protect against prostate cancer and Alzheimer's disease.

Recommended food sources: mustard greens, boiled spinach, wheat germ, nuts, green leafy vegetables, fortified cereals, whole grains, fish, peanut butter, sunflower seeds, turnip greens, almonds, collard greens, kale, papaya, olives, olive oils, vegetable oils, bell peppers, Brussels sprouts, kiwi fruit, tomatoes, blueberries, and steamed broccoli.

Signs of shortage include: digestive system problems; tingling or loss of sensation in arms, hands, legs, or feet; liver or gallbladder problems; and neurological problems due to poor nerve conduction.

4. **Vitamin K.** This nutrient is needed for proper bone formation and helps your body transport calcium, which is used in blood clotting, thus it is prescribed to prevent excessive bleeding. It facilitates blood coagulation, aids in maintaining strong bones and healthy hearts, and increases blood flow to the digestive tract. It helps to protect against osteoporosis and hardening of the arteries, and prevents oxidative cell damage.

    Recommended food sources: parsley, olive oil, soybean oil, canola oil, boiled kale, spinach, mustard greens, turnip greens, Swiss chard, collard greens, romaine lettuce, steamed broccoli, Brussels sprouts, cabbage, asparagus, celery, black pepper, green beans, cauliflower, tomatoes, green peas, carrots, bell peppers, squash, avocados, soy beans, cranberries, strawberries, papaya, and kidney beans.

Signs of shortage include: excessive bruising and bleeding, digestive system problems, and liver or gallbladder problems.

Minerals

While vitamins are organic, minerals are different because they are inorganic in nature. Minerals do not provide your body with an energy source, but they play a vital role in several physiological functions. These include involvement in the functioning of the nervous system, in cellular reactions, in maintaining water balance, and in the structural systems of your body. They play important roles in sustaining life and maintaining optimal health. They are essential nutrients. Body-building minerals serve as the structure of bones and teeth. Some minerals help to maintain the balance of acids and bases in your body. Minerals are also important in the transmission of nerve impulses, and some are necessary for muscle connection and relaxation. Minerals help vitamins and other nutrients to work more efficiently in your body. If you eat a balanced and varied diet, you should be able to take in minerals in all of the amounts you need to stay healthy. This should include a lot of fresh fruits and vegetables and protein sources, like meat or beans. If you don't eat a balanced diet, then taking a mineral supplement may be necessary. Because minerals have simple structures, usually just one or more molecules of an element, they are not easily destroyed during food preparation. They are stable substances that do not break down at temperatures used in cooking. In the case of food minerals, more is not better. You can get ill from taking too much of any food mineral. (The same is true for various vitamins and herbs.)

Of the seventeen essential minerals, there is a great variance regarding the amounts that are needed each day. For this reason minerals are divided into two classes. The first class of minerals is macro-minerals, which are needed in greater quantities that range from milligrams to grams. Your body needs one hundred milligrams or more of each of these each day. The second class of minerals is micro-minerals, which are needed in smaller quantities, generally between a microgram and a milligram. Your body needs less than one hundred milligrams of any micro-mineral each day. Dietary requirements have not yet been established for some minerals. The health benefits and food sources of macro-minerals and micro-minerals are listed below.

Macro-minerals

Macro-minerals are needed in larger amounts in your body, one hundred milligrams or more per day.

1. **Calcium.** This is an important mineral for bone and tooth structure, blood clotting, and nerve transmission. Almost all calcium is found in bones. Calcium is responsible for forming your bones and teeth and helps prevent osteoporosis. It is required for muscle contraction, blood vessel expansion and contraction, secretion of hormones and enzymes, and transmitting impulses throughout the nervous system. Other important functions include aiding coagulation of the blood and the contraction of muscles, supporting the strength and firmness of your skeleton, impacting cardiac action, transforming light to electrical impulses in your retina, and aiding chemical reactions in your body and milk production.

   Recommended food sources: milk, cheese, yogurt, collard greens, spinach, chard, mustard greens, broccoli, green peppers, dried beans and peas, navy beans, soy beans, split peas, fortified orange juice, almonds, Brazil nuts, breads, cereals, salmon, sardines, Brussels sprouts, okra, and baked beans.

Signs of shortage include: frequent bone fractures, muscle pain or spasms, tingling or numbness in your hands or feet, bone deformities, and growth retardation in children.

2. **Phosphorus.** This is the second most abundant mineral in your body, and 85 percent of it is found in your bones. The main purpose of phosphorus is building strong bones and teeth; however, practically every cell in your body uses it. Phosphorus works in concert with calcium; a healthy balance of calcium to phosphorus is two to one. It may be beneficial in the treatment of fractures, brittle bones, rickets, and teeth and gum disorders. Phosphorus protects and strengthens all cell membranes and assists other nutrients and chemicals in their bodily processes. It is needed for healthy nerve impulses, normal kidney functioning, and the utilization of carbohydrates, fats, and proteins for growth, maintenance, and repair of cells, and for energy production. Without phosphorus you would be unable to move. Phosphorus helps maintain heart regularity, provides energy, and aids in the metabolizing of fats and starches. It also aids in growth and body repair, reduces arthritis pain, and it may even help in cancer prevention.

Recommended food sources: milk, yogurt, cottage cheese, hamburger, tuna, sunflower seeds, peanuts, peanut butter, sweet potatoes, tomato paste, baked potato, tomato puree, prune juice, carrot juice, bananas, tomato juice, orange juice, cantaloupe, kidney beans, whole wheat, noodles, rice, potatoes, corn, peas, and broccoli.

Signs of shortage include: weak or fragile bones and teeth, fatigue, weakness, lack of appetite, joint pain and stiffness, confusion, lethargy, and a susceptibility to infections. A shortage can also lead to rickets, arthritis, and tooth decay.

3. **Magnesium.** This mineral is important for maintaining a healthy heart, and it can help to prevent heart disease and stroke. Magnesium is a constituent of bones and is present in all of your body cells. Magnesium helps in maintaining blood pressure by regulating blood sugar levels, is vital for maintaining a healthy heart, helps prevent abnormal blood clotting in the heart, maintains proper muscle function, and keeps the muscles relaxed. It helps in absorbing calcium and potassium and is necessary for the proper functioning of the nervous system. Magnesium has a relaxing effect on the airways in the lungs and is needed for more than three hundred biochemical reactions in your body. Magnesium supports a healthy immune system, keeps bones strong, and is involved in energy metabolism and protein synthesis. More than 50 percent of Americans do not get the recommended daily allowance (RDA) of magnesium in their diets. It is the fourth most prominent mineral in the body, and 50 percent is found in your bones.

Recommended food sources: halibut, tuna, bananas, oat bran, brown rice, prune juice, low-fat yogurt, almonds, Brazil nuts, cashews, baked beans, black beans, lima beans, kidney beans, navy beans, pinto beans, broccoli, chickpeas, lentils, peas, pumpkin, spinach, squash, sweet potatoes, tomato paste, walleye, potatoes, okra, and haddock.

Signs of shortage include: nervousness, anxiety, agitated sleep and frequent awakening, leg cramps, migraines, fatigue, loss of appetite, depression, nausea, vomiting, and high blood pressure.

4. **Sodium.** A safe intake of this essential nutrient is between 0.9 to 2.3 grams per day. Sodium is needed for normal body function. It maintains the right balance of fluids in your body, helps transmit nerve impulses, and influences the contraction and relaxation of your muscles.

    Recommended food sources: Sodium is found naturally in many foods and can be added to foods in the form of salt or other sodium-containing substances. Rock salt and sea salt are almost entirely sodium chloride. The issue with sodium is usually not whether you get *enough* sodium in your diet but rather whether you have *too much.*

    Consequences of excess of sodium in your blood: When your kidneys can't excrete enough sodium, the excess starts to accumulate in your body. This excess then leaks to the surrounding tissues, causing swelling, especially in the ankles and feet. Because sodium attracts and holds water, high sodium concentration in your body will lead to an increase in the blood volume. Increased blood volume makes your heart work harder to move more blood through your blood vessels, which increases pressure in your arteries. Excess sodium in your blood is very serious and can lead to organ failure and death. High blood pressure is rarely seen in those who consume less than 1.2 grams of sodium per day.

5. **Chloride.** Normal values for the total amount of chloride in your blood range from 98 to 106 milliequivalents (one thousandth of a gram equivalent of a chemical element) per liter.

    Recommended food sources: It is found in table salt or sea salt as sodium chloride and is also found in many vegetables. Foods with higher amounts of chloride include seaweed, rye, tomatoes, celery, lettuce, and olives. Potassium chloride is found in most foods and is usually the main ingredient in salt substitutes.

Signs of excess chloride in your blood include: dehydration, vomiting, diarrhea, excessive urination, and severe burns.

Signs of shortage include: kidney disease, uncontrolled diabetes, congestive heart failure, cirrhosis of the liver, and very high levels of protein, triglycerides, or glucose in your blood.

6. **Potassium.** The normal functioning of all cells, muscle function, the transmission of nerve impulses, prevention of excess fluid retention, and the metabolism of carbohydrates and proteins all require potassium. This mineral aids in muscle contraction. It assists in maintaining the appropriate levels of fluids in your cells and monitors the balance of electrolytes in your cells. It may also prevent high blood pressure. Potassium enables your body to convert glucose into energy, and it helps prevent kidney stones. Your kidneys maintain the right amount of potassium in your body. If your kidneys are not functioning properly, you need to limit the foods you eat which cause high levels of potassium in your blood.

Recommended food sources: apricots, bananas, baked potatoes, sweet potatoes, yogurt, prune juice, carrot juice, tomato juice, spinach, lentils, tomato puree, beans, milk, Brussels sprouts, black-eyed peas, Brazil nuts, cantaloupe, raisins, prunes, tomato sauce, tomato juice, orange juice, and chickpeas.

Signs of excess potassium include: irregular heartbeats and heart attack, weakness, numbness, low blood pressure, kidney disease, muscle spasms or cramps, joint and back pain, bladder infections, poor immune system function, anxiety, insomnia, irritability, and impotence. Cancer risk also increases when potassium levels are too high.

Symptoms of shortage include: irregular and/or rapid heartbeat, high blood pressure, stroke, kidney disease, asthma, muscle spasms, weakness, water retention, high blood sugar, liver disease, weight gain, fatigue, and impotence.

Micro-minerals

Micro-minerals are minerals required by the body in relatively small amounts of less than one hundred milligrams per day.

1. **Iron.** Iron is vital to life. Every cell in the human body contains it. Oxygenation of tissues and cells is accomplished by iron in red blood cells that carry oxygenated blood throughout your body and pick up carbon dioxide to be excreted. (Iron makes up an important part of hemoglobin, the substance in your blood that carries oxygen throughout your body.) Iron enhances immune system functioning, produces energy, and increases oxygen distribution throughout the body. It is important for muscle protein. Iron carries oxygen to muscles, helping them to function properly. Iron helps increase your resistance to stress and disease.

    Recommended food sources: beef, tuna, salmon, liver, eggs, broccoli, turkey, sardines, poultry, fish, cooked beans, lentils, dried beans, peas, iron-fortified cereals, baked potato with skin, canned asparagus, pumpkin seeds, bread, pasta products, spinach, mustard greens, kale, chard, dried fruits, nuts, and seeds. Tannins (found in teas), calcium, polyphenols and phytates found in legumes, and whole grains can decrease the absorption of iron. Meat proteins and vitamin C will increase iron absorption.[2]

Signs of iron shortage include: anemia, weight loss, paleness, intestinal disorders, panting, palpitation, general fatigue, and a shortage of red blood cells.

2. **Zinc.** This micro-mineral stimulates the activity of approximately one hundred enzymes, substances that promote biochemical activity in your body. Zinc is an essential mineral that is found in every cell in your body. It supports a healthy immune system, is needed for wound healing, helps protect your body against viruses, activates white blood cells to fight infections, helps maintain your senses of taste and smell, and is needed for DNA synthesis. It supports normal growth and development during pregnancy, childhood, and adolescence. It also helps stabilize blood sugar and metabolic rate.

Recommended food sources? Lean beef tenderloin, venison, sesame seeds, pumpkin seeds, low-fat yogurt, green peas, calf liver, spinach, mushrooms, black-eyed peas, Brazil nuts, cashews, chickpeas, eggs, legumes, lima beans, oats, pecans, sardines, turkey, poultry, beans, whole grains, fortified cereals, and dairy products.

Signs of shortage include: growth retardation, hair loss, diarrhea, impotence, eye and skin lesions, loss of appetite, weight loss, delayed healing of wounds, impaired sense of taste or smell, depression, frequent colds, infections, and mental lethargy.

3. **Selenium.** This important antioxidant protects cells from free radical damage. It is beneficial for treating and preventing allergies, arthritis, chronic fatigue syndrome, heart disease, macular degeneration, stroke, and various types of cancer. A deficiency of selenium is linked to AIDS and miscarriages. It helps to combat viruses, protects against heart disease and circulatory diseases, enables your thyroid to produce thyroid hormone, helps lower the risk of joint inflammation, helps male potency, and supports healthy eyes, skin, and hair.

   Recommended food sources: Brazil nuts, kidney beans, turkey, sardines, wheat flour, whole wheat spaghetti, egg noodles, liver, whole-meal bread, mackerel, wheat germ, bran, tuna fish, onions, tomatoes, mushrooms, cod, snapper, halibut, salmon, barley, and broccoli.

   Signs of shortage include: Weakness or pain in your muscles, discoloration of your hair and skin, and whitening of your fingernail beds.

4. **Copper.** This micro-mineral helps fight against heart attacks and strokes, supports healthy immune system function, helps your body utilize iron, keeps your thyroid gland functioning properly, preserves the myelin sheaths that surround and protect your nerves, and maintains the health of your bones and connective tissues. Copper is a catalyst in the formation of hemoglobin and acts on your body to remove free radicals that cause heart disease and certain cancers. Copper can alleviate some arthritis pain as well.

   Recommended food sources: calf liver, barley, soy beans, chickpeas, navy beans, sunflower seeds, sesame seeds, lean beef, almonds, avocados, green leafy vegetables, barley, broccoli, seafood, beets, pecans, rye, butter, carrots, whole wheat, raisins, cereals, oats, potatoes, mushrooms, radishes, Brazil nuts, cashew nuts, butter beans, lentils, walnuts, peanuts, whole-meal bread, and mackerel.

Signs of shortage include: iron-deficiency anemia, easily ruptured blood vessels, bone and joint problems, elevated LDL (bad) cholesterol, reduced HDL (good) cholesterol, frequent infections, loss of hair or skin color, fatigue and weakness, difficulty breathing, irregular heartbeat, skin sores, and dry skin.

5. Manganese. In addition to its antioxidant, free-radical-fighting properties, manganese is important for proper food digestion and normal bone structure. It helps your body convert protein and fat to energy. It also helps to maintain healthy reproductive, nervous, and immune systems, helps your body synthesize fatty acids and cholesterol, promotes optimal functioning of your thyroid gland, maintains the health of your nerves, and aids in blood sugar regulation. It is involved in blood clotting and the formation of cartilage and lubricating fluid in the joints. It is stored predominantly in the bones, liver, kidney, and pancreas.

    Recommended food sources: avocados, nuts and seeds, tea, raisins, pineapple, spinach, broccoli, oranges, beans, rye, oats, blueberries, apples, celery, egg yolks, walnuts, apricots, brown rice, chickpeas, spinach, dried peas, olives, blackberries, and green leafy vegetables.

    Signs of shortage include: infertility, bone malformation, weakness, seizures, atherosclerosis, confusion, convulsions, eye problems, nausea, vomiting, skin rash, loss of hair color, dizziness, hearing loss, reproductive system difficulties, heart disorders, high cholesterol, hypertension, irritability, memory loss, muscle contractions, pancreatic damage, profuse perspiration, rapid pulse, tooth grinding, tremors, and osteoporosis.

6. **Chromium.** This regulator of blood sugar levels has been used to treat diabetes. It is the glucose tolerance factor that stimulates insulin activity. Chromium controls your uptake of glucose by the muscles and organs, stimulates glucose metabolism, controls blood cholesterol levels, controls fat levels in the blood, reduces atherosclerosis, stimulates the synthesis of proteins, increases resistance to infection, and controls hunger pains.

Recommended food sources: liver, whole-grain cereals, rye bread, potatoes, whole-wheat bread, eggs, butter, apples, Swiss cheese, brown rice, fresh fruits and vegetables, meat, cheese, Brewer's yeast, molasses, mushrooms, raw onions, romaine lettuce, tomatoes, and egg yolk.

Signs of shortage include: diabetes, hypoglycemia, fatigue, mood swings, insulin resistance, high blood cholesterol, atherosclerosis, and loss of sugar in the urine.

7. **Molybdenum.** This micro-mineral is thought to aid in the metabolism of fats and carbohydrates. Molybdenum is involved in protein synthesis, is vital for the utilization of iron, protects against cancer, prevents anemia, aids in the formation of uric acid, promotes a feeling of general well-being, helps prevent sexual impotence in men, and helps to prevent tooth decay.

Recommended food sources: canned beans, wheat germ, whole wheat, liver, whole grains, black beans, lima beans, peanuts, kidney beans, navy beans, black-eyed peas, chestnuts, cashews, yogurt, eggs, legumes, peas, and dark green leafy vegetables.

Signs of shortage include: irregular heartbeat, irritability, and an inability to produce uric acid.

8. **Boron.** Boron helps to maintain the levels of minerals and hormones that are needed for bone health, may aid in the prevention of calcium loss to help prevent osteoporosis, and raises testosterone levels in men to allow for the building of muscle. It facilitates various enzyme reactions for your body, regulates estrogen levels, promotes proper mental functioning, and alertness and keeps cell walls strong so that proper transfer of nutrients can occur.

   Recommended food sources: pears, prunes, raisins, tomatoes, apples, almonds, dried apricots, avocados, bananas, red kidney beans, peanut butter, honey, wheat bran, Brazil nuts, broccoli, carrots, celery, red grapes, cashew nuts, chickpeas, and dates.

   Signs of shortage include: depression, problems metabolizing calcium, magnesium, and phosphorus, and increased effects of stress on the body.

To better understand the nutrition deficiencies that exist in the typical American diet, I have listed some data below regarding some of the vitamins and minerals that we typically consume in amounts well below the standard necessary for optimal health. When there are nutritional deficiencies, there is an increased risk of illness and disease.

- Required amounts of fiber may be lacking in many diets. Men should be eating approximately thirty-eight grams of fiber each day, and women should be consuming twenty-five grams per day[3]

- It has been estimated that 56 percent of Americans are not getting enough magnesium in their diets. This nutrient is critical for a healthy circulatory system and healthy bones.[4]
- Approximately 70 percent of Americans do not consume enough calcium daily.[5] Calcium is critical in maintaining strong bones, supporting nerve and muscle function, and maintaining a healthy blood pressure.
- Potassium helps support proper nerve and muscle function, maintain a healthy blood pressure, and regulate body fluids, yet it is estimated that 97 percent of Americans aren't getting enough potassium.[6]
- It has been estimated that 93 percent of Americans are not getting enough vitamin E in their diets.[7] This nutrient is critical in boosting your immune system.
- Over 30 percent of Americans do not get enough vitamin C.[8] This is another vitamin that helps protect your body from disease by boosting your immune system.
- It has been estimated that 44 percent of Americans do not get enough vitamin A in their diets. Vitamin A plays a key role in supporting a healthy immune system as well as in preserving eyesight and supporting healthy skin.[9]

All three of the vitamins mentioned above—E, C, and A—are found in certain fruits and vegetables. A strong immune system is critical in preventing disease and infection. A healthy strategy for maintaining good health is to make sure that you include a minimum of five to eight servings of fruits and/or vegetables in your diet each day.

Though supplementation of vitamins and minerals can be very desirable for many people, it is important to understand the reasons for taking the supplements as well as the appropriate quantities. Due to certain health situations and conditions, it is advisable that certain supplements be taken under a doctor's supervision; some supplements can cause adverse reactions and become detrimental to your health.

You should never take any supplement unless you are fully aware of the purpose and the likely impact on your health. Though I have been taking supplements for more than ten years, with no adverse effects, every person—and his or her health—is unique.

If it is your goal to be healthy and enhance your quality of life, it is imperative to take an inventory of the food choices that you make on a day-to-day basis. We all need a working knowledge of which nutrients our bodies utilize to operate efficiently, and we need to know where to get those nutrients so that we are not at the mercy of advertising and cultural choices. It is particularly important to have this information because of the prevalence of fast food meals and processed foods that lack the nutrients essential to sustaining a healthy body. When your body is not being fed proper nutrients, you have opened the door for disease. Over time, your body will break down, and you will have health problems. In the case of vitamins and minerals, what you don't know *will* hurt you!

The nutritional guidelines in the United States have gone through many changes since the recommended daily allowances (RDA) were first established in 1941. Recommendations have gone from the minimum amount of nutrients needed to prevent serious diseases to amounts that are more likely to promote and support optimal health. If you are curious about nutritional recommendations, a brief discussion of the history of these recommendations follows.

The recommended daily allowances (RDA) were established during World War II by a committee funded by the National Academy of Sciences for the purpose of investigating nutrition issues that might impact national defense. The committee was renamed the Food and Nutrition Board in 1941. It was the committee's task to determine a set of recommendations to define a desirable standard daily allowance of each type of nutrient for the armed forces, as well as civilian and overseas populations who might need food relief. The final set of RDA guidelines was accepted in 1941. The Food and Nutrition Board revised the RDA guidelines every five to ten years.

In 1968 the recommended daily intake (RDI) was introduced. The nutritional recommendations were still based upon the older recommendations of the RDAs. The guidelines of the RDI were based on nutrient levels, which were considered (at the time they were defined) to be sufficient to meet the requirements of nearly all (97 to 98 percent) healthy individuals of both sexes in each stage of life. The RDI replaced the RDA and is used today in the United States and Canada to determine the daily nutritional values on food labels.

In 1997, the United States Department of Agriculture (USDA) created newer guidelines called the Dietary Reference Intake (DRI) to broaden the existing guidelines of the recommended daily intake (RDI). The new DRI guidelines categorized nutritional intake at four different levels: estimated average requirements (EAR), recommended dietary allowances (RDA), adequate intake (AI), and tolerable upper intake (UL). These nutritional recommendations came from the Institute of Medicine (IOM) of the National Academy of Sciences.

The optimal daily intake (ODI) nutritional recommendations evolved from the idea that you should consume nutrients at levels that a consensus of scientific studies has shown promote optimal health and vitality. The ODI recommendations for many of the nutrients are much greater than those of the RDA. The only possible means of attaining these optimal levels is through vitamin and mineral supplementation, because it would be difficult to eat enough food to reach the recommended levels. For the purpose of this chapter, I will contrast the nutritional daily recommendations of both the recommended daily intake (minimum levels) and the optimal daily intakes (desirable levels) for review. Both of these sources make recommendations for vitamins and minerals. (See the comparison chart of recommended daily intakes and optimal daily intakes[10] in the appendix to become familiar with the names of the vitamins and minerals and identify the quantities that are recommended for optimal health benefits.

Chapter 8:

Do I Really Need to Exercise? (The Answer Is Yes!)

If you are serious about maintaining good health, it is absolutely necessary to exercise. Good nutrition and exercise go hand in hand in maintaining a healthy body. There are many positive health benefits in beginning and maintaining an exercise program. Consider some of these main health benefits:

- **Exercise helps to prevent diseases.** Exercise reduces the risk of heart disease, cancer, high blood pressure, diabetes, and other diseases. It is essential in maintaining cardiorespiratory fitness.
- **Exercise controls body weight.** Being overweight is a risk factor for a number of diseases, and exercise is your key to weight control because it burns calories. Your body is meant to move, and this movement speeds up your metabolism, which is essential in weight control.
- **Exercise increases your stamina.** The energy expended during exercise improves your stamina by training your body to become more efficient and use less energy to complete a given amount of work. It promotes the conditioning necessary to improve your heart rate and

breathing rate so that you return to your normal rates faster than if you were not fit.

- **Exercise strengthens and tones your muscles, bones, and ligaments.** Exercise increases your strength and endurance. Posture can also be improved through exercise, and muscles become more firm and toned as a result of participating in an exercise program.
- **Exercise improves your flexibility.** Stretching exercises promote flexibility, which allows you to bend, reach, and twist without a reduction in range. Improved flexibility reduces the chance of injury and improves balance and coordination.
- **Exercise has emotional benefits.** Exercising helps reduce your stress and promotes a positive mind-set.
- **Exercise helps you to sleep better.** Lack of adequate sleep is a risk factor for unwanted health problems.

The expression "Use it or lose it" is accurate. Inactivity is as much of a health risk factor as smoking![1] You need to do the most difficult part first—get started! You will then be on your way to a healthier lifestyle.

For the purpose of this chapter, I am going to recommend a general fitness program that will provide an overall balance that is sustainable throughout your life. If followed over a period of time, the program will provide an adequate level of physical fitness. It is one that I recommend for those who have not been actively involved in a physical fitness program. When your level of physical fitness increases and you desire more variety in your exercise program, you may need to make some changes in your exercise routine. It is good to change exercise programs every few months to avoid staleness and to utilize a variety of exercises that impact different muscles. Your focus now is simply to get started!

In this chapter I will define certain terminology and explain how this sample program should be implemented. For better understanding, I will first present each program component separately. Then, at the end, I will provide an overview regarding the program as a whole. There are four major components that I believe should be part of any exercise program. I am confident that these components will be more than adequate for many of you. The workout components that I focus on are aerobic exercise, walking, weight-resistance exercises, and stretching.

> *Caution:* Before beginning an exercise program it is important to make sure that you have no medical limitations. A physical exam by a physician can be helpful in determining what you can do and what you should not do when participating in an exercise program.

If you are free from any physical restrictions, I recommend an exercise program that includes at least three aerobic workouts and three weight-resistance workouts every week. These intentional workouts should last between thirty and sixty minutes each day. The aerobic and weight-resistance workouts should be on alternate days. For instance, if you do aerobics on Monday, Wednesday, and Friday, then weight-resistance workouts should be scheduled on Tuesday, Thursday, and Saturday. Sunday can be a rest day or an optional light aerobic workout day (walking or bicycle riding). Keep in mind that these are the scheduled, intentional workouts. In addition to these scheduled workouts, moving more is an important addition to make to your daily activity. This includes things such as walking rather than driving or riding the bus or train, taking the stairs instead of using an elevator, working in the yard, and doing activities that require you to move more than your present habits dictate.

Aerobics

What is aerobics? The American College of Sports Medicine defines aerobic exercise as any activity that uses large muscle groups, can be maintained continuously, and is rhythmic in nature.[2] Aerobics is also defined as exercise that increases the need for oxygen. Aerobic exercises often go by other names including cardiovascular exercises and cardio.

The Benefits

Some of the benefits of aerobic exercise are listed below.

- **Reduces body fat and improves your ability to control your body weight.** Exercise burns calories. Spending just fifteen minutes per day to walk one mile will burn one hundred extra calories each day. This would result in a loss of ten pounds in one year if you kept your eating exactly the same.
- **Improves the function of your heart and lungs.** Exercise forces the chest to make extensive inhalations and exhalations. Over time this causes your maximum lung capacity to increase. This improves lung function by facilitating the exchange of oxygen and carbon dioxide. Your heart responds to exercise demands by becoming bigger and stronger. The heart moves blood through your body with fewer contractions, and the rest of your muscles in your body receive oxygen more quickly.
- **Decreases your LDL (bad) cholesterol.** Since exercise helps to burn up fat in your body and cholesterol is a type of fat, then cholesterol is burned up during exercise. This causes cholesterol levels to decrease through exercise. Any kind of exercise is helpful in lowering cholesterol levels.
- **Improves your HDL (good) cholesterol.** Though researchers do not know exactly how exercise increases good cholesterol (HDL), current research has shown that as little as thirty minutes of aerobic exercise five days per week raises HDL cholesterol. According to the Mayo clinic, just two months of aerobic exercise can increase your HDL cholesterol by about 5 percent. Losing unhealthy body fat is another by-product of

aerobic exercise. When this happens there are significant increases in HDL cholesterol.

- **Improves your oxygen capacity.** Exercise increases your rate of breathing and your body's demand for oxygen. This demand on your heart and lungs increases your lung's capacity for work.
- **Increases your blood supply to your muscles.** When you exercise, the blood vessels in your muscles dilate, and this increases the blood flow. This increase in blood flow delivers more oxygenated blood to the working muscles.
- **Improves the efficiency of your muscles to use oxygen.** If you exercise more than a couple of minutes, your body needs to get oxygen to the muscles, or the muscles will stop working. Because exercise causes your heart to get stronger, your heart can deliver more oxygen to your muscles. As a result, your muscles become more efficient at using the oxygen.
- **Lowers your resting heart rate.** Aerobic training causes the heart wall to increase in thickness, which makes your heart a more powerful pump. This allows your heart to pump a greater volume of blood. Your resting heart rate will then decrease because your heart can still keep up with the demand for oxygen. Lance Armstrong, multiple Tour de France cycling champion, had his resting heart rate measured at thirty-two beats per minute. The average resting heart rate is between sixty to eighty beats per minute.
- **Improves glucose tolerance and reduces insulin resistance.** Regular exercise primes your cells for activity. To get the energy that you need for exercise, your body uses insulin to move sugar and fat into cells, where they are burned as fuel. With the increase in insulin activity, sugar levels in the blood decrease. With less sugar in your blood, your body produces less insulin and becomes more responsive to both sugar and insulin.

Insulin sensitivity (the opposite of insulin resistance) goes up, and that's good. The loss of unhealthy weight from exercise further increases insulin sensitivity. This is one reason why the American Heart Association recommends a minimum of thirty minutes of exercise five days per week. This will promote weight loss and the improvement of insulin sensitivity.

- **Reduces your resting blood pressure (systolic and diastolic).** Regular aerobic exercise strengthens the heart and increases the stroke volume of your heart. Your stroke volume is the amount of blood that is pumped by the left ventricle of your heart in one contraction. The more blood you pump, the less often your heart has to pump. The less often your heart pumps, the lower the pressure is in your veins and arteries. Thus, increasing your stroke volume through aerobic exercise reduces your resting blood pressure.

- **Decreases the effects of anxiety, tension, and depression.** This happens in a number of ways, including releasing feel-good brain chemicals (neurotransmitters and endorphins), reducing immune system chemicals that can worsen depression, and increasing body temperature, which can have a calming effect on the body. Other emotional benefits are the self-confidence gained by meeting exercise goals and challenges. Exercise can also take your mind off your worries by serving as a distraction from negative thoughts that feed anxiety and depression. Exercise is a positive way to manage depression because it adds to the health of your body. It can also provide an opportunity for more social interaction by putting you in settings where you can socialize and meet other people.

- **Increases your threshold for muscle fatigue.** Your muscle fatigue threshold is commonly referred to as anaerobic threshold or lactate threshold. When your short-term energy stores become depleted and lactic acid begins to accumulate in the muscles, exercise soon comes to a halt. Let's say you were to engage in an all-out sprint. Lactic acid would begin to accumulate after your energy stores became depleted. You would then be unable to continue sprinting. This occurs when the oxygen demands of the working muscles are not met. Exercise will cause your aerobic and anaerobic endurance to improve over time, and your body will become more efficient at producing the energy that you need. Exercise loads that were very difficult when you first began your exercise program will become much easier as your threshold improves.[3]

These physical and emotional benefits are too significant and important to ignore. Aerobic exercise is another preventive tool that contributes to optimum health and should be included in any balanced exercise program.

The Components

A complete aerobic workout includes a warm-up, the aerobic workout, and a cool-down period after the workout. There are four important factors to consider when setting up an aerobic workout:

1. **Frequency:** the number of days per week that you do aerobic exercises.
2. **Duration:** the length of your workouts.
3. **Type:** the particular aerobic exercise that you choose to engage in.
4. **Intensity:** how difficult the activity is. This should be determined by the percentage of your maximum heart rate achieved during your workout.

First, you need to determine frequency. My recommendation is three days per week. Every activity utilizes different muscles. You should not work the same muscles by doing the same types of activities on consecutive days because muscles need time to rest and heal. A day of rest in between a specific type of activity will allow you time for healing and prevent overuse injuries. Keeping all this in mind, you can decide to do aerobic workouts with a frequency of three days per week, on Monday, Wednesday, and Friday.

Second, you need to determine duration. You can choose the same amount of time for each aerobic workout, or for variety, you can alter the length of your workouts. For example, each Monday, you could do a twenty-five-minute aerobic workout; on Wednesday, a thirty-five-minute workout; and on Friday, you could select a twenty-minute aerobic workout. Regardless, the workout duration should last between twenty and sixty minutes. It should be noted that shorter is not necessarily easier because you can work out with greater intensity for twenty minutes than for sixty minutes. The purpose of changing the length of time is for variety and also to allow for different levels of intensity.

The third variable to consider is the actual type of aerobic workout. Some examples of aerobic exercise include running, swimming, cycling, EFX, jumping rope, walking briskly, cross-country skiing, jogging, stair climbing, rollerblading, rowing, taking aerobics classes, and other exercises that increase the oxygen that is available to the working muscles. For instance, on Mondays you could jog; on Wednesdays you could swim laps; and on Fridays you could choose cycling. As long as the frequency, duration, and intensity are appropriate, you can change the aerobic workout. One major advantage of changing activities is that different activities require the use of different muscle groups. A variety of different activities can also help combat boredom.

The fourth component of an aerobic workout is intensity. Intensity should be determined by two main factors: fitness level and age. Your maximum heart rate is usually computed by taking the number 220 and subtracting your age.[4] If you are fifty years old, for example, then your maximum heart rate would be 170 (220 − 50 = 170). The younger you are, the higher your maximum heart rate will be. During your aerobic workout, you should maintain a heart rate between 60 and 85 percent of your maximum heart rate.[5] (Different sources have varied recommendations as to the minimum heart rate during aerobic exercises. Typically, these percentages range from 50 to 85 percent or from 60 to 85 percent. Regardless, these percentages determine the range of your intensity.)

Your present fitness level will determine the level of intensity that you can maintain. Using the same example above, if your maximum heart rate is 170, then during your aerobic workout, you should maintain a heart rate of 60 to 85 percent of 170 beats per minute, that is, between 102 and 145 beats per minute. This is the range that you should strive to maintain during the duration of your aerobic workout. If you are more fit, you will be able to maintain a heart rate closer to 145 beats per minute for the duration of the workout without overtraining. If you are not as fit, it will be necessary to reduce the intensity closer to 102 beats per minute (60 percent) until you become more fit. It should never be your goal to work out beyond your physical capacity. Always start an aerobic exercise program at a moderate level and build up to more challenging workouts when your fitness level increases.

If you are unable to maintain a heart rate between 60 to 85 percent of your maximum heart rate without exceptional strain for the duration of an aerobic workout, you are not yet ready to do aerobic exercise. When your physical condition will not allow you to engage in aerobic exercises, there are two options:

1. Do aerobic exercises at a lower intensity until your body becomes fit enough to exercise at the recommended intensity.
2. Begin with a walking program in place of the aerobic exercises. If this is necessary, I recommend thirty to sixty minutes of walking each day. Walking is less intense than aerobics and is often the best option if you are at an unhealthy body weight or suffer from a physical limitation that makes aerobics an unwise choice. If walking is not desirable due to problems with knees or hips, exercise in a swimming pool is a good alternative. Aerobic pool activities offer the added

benefit of decreasing the shock to the knee, ankle, and hip areas.

Doing nothing is never the best option! Your focus should always be on what you *can* do rather than on what you cannot do.

Walking

When you are too unfit to engage in even a less intense aerobic exercise plan, I recommend starting with a walking program in place of aerobics. Walking lacks the intensity of aerobics, but it does not lack in physical benefits. Consider the following potential benefits of adding walking to your exercise program:

- Managing your body weight
- Controlling blood pressure
- Reducing the risk of heart attack
- Lowering LDL (bad) cholesterol
- Increasing HDL (good) cholesterol
- Reducing the risk of type 2 diabetes
- Reducing the risk of breast cancer
- Reducing the risk of a hip fracture
- Relieving arthritis
- Reducing the risk of a stroke
- Improving your sleep
- Relieving back pain
- Preventing depression
- Reducing the risk of osteoporosis[6]

The benefits are many, and the dangers are few. Regardless of your fitness level, if you are able, walking should be part of your overall fitness program. If you use a pedometer to gauge your walking, I recommend a minimum of ten thousand steps per day; this is just a target point to assure that you are getting a minimum amount of movement each day. The speed that you walk will be dependent upon your present level of fitness. Your goal should be to complete it without undo health risk. You should always start out gradually and increase the pace of your walk. If there are any questions regarding your readiness to perform any exercise program, you should seek the advice of your physician.

If you do aerobic workouts, this does not mean that you should exclude walking. To increase your fitness level you will need to increase your movement. Even though I complete very intense aerobic workouts four days per week, I believe walking is still a valuable form of exercise for me because it provides additional movement. Since there is not enough movement in our culture, any type of movement is important. Walking is like the frosting on the cake for those who do aerobics. It is the one exercise that most people can do every day without overtraining.

Weight Resistance

Weight-resistance workouts are also called weight training or strength training. The goal of this type of training is to increase muscular strength, muscular endurance, or muscular power. My recommendation is that these workouts should focus upon both muscular strength and muscular endurance. Muscular power workouts are generally reserved for those who engage in athletic competitions that require muscular power. This is not necessary for those of you whose goal is to become physically fit.

The Benefits

Like aerobic exercises, weight-resistance exercises represent many potential health benefits, so many that I believe they must be included in any well-balanced exercise program. Some of the potential benefits of weight-training exercises include:

- Improving posture
- Relief of lower back pain
- Protection of your internal organs

- Increasing your resting metabolism
- Lowering blood pressure
- Preventing osteoporosis
- Increasing HDL (good) cholesterol
- Decreasing total cholesterol
- Increasing the breakdown of fat
- Improving sleeping patterns
- Increasing the strength of bones
- Reducing the risk of many debilitating diseases
- Reducing stress and increasing emotional well-being[7]

The Components

There are a number of components to consider when planning a weight-resistance exercise program. They are:

1. **Frequency:** the number of days each week that you do weight-resistance exercises. My recommendation is three days per week, on days when you are not doing aerobic workouts. For example, you may want to do aerobics on Monday, Wednesday, and Friday; so, your weight-resistance workouts would be on Tuesday, Thursday, and Saturday.

2. **Duration:** the length of each weight-resistance workout. I recommend between thirty and forty-five minutes for each workout.

3. **Type:** the method used to complete a weight-resistance workout. Weight-resistance exercises can be accomplished with dumbbells, barbells, resistance machines, bands, or rubber tubing or your own body weight.

4. **Repetitions:** the number of times that you complete a particular exercise before stopping. Initially, I recommend twelve repetitions of each set. For example, if you do three sets of an exercise, you would do twelve repetitions three times. You would do one set of twelve repetitions, rest, than do another set of twelve repetitions,

rest, and then do a final set of twelve repetitions. This can be adjusted after a period of time. There is a benefit to doing higher repetitions on one workout and, the next time the workout is completed, changing to lower, heavier repetitions. Variety is good. Change is good. It helps to prevent staleness and boredom. It also allows a balance of exercises that target both muscular strength and muscular endurance. In general, the higher repetitions are performed to build muscular endurance. Lower repetitions with heavier weights are performed to develop strength and power. Be aware that fewer repetitions, that involve heavier weights, increase the possibility of injury. This is due to the fact that you may tend to compromise proper lifting technique to accommodate the heavier weights that are used. The key to avoiding injury in weight-resistance exercises is to lift properly and to select resistances that allow you to lift with proper form.

5. **Rest period:** the length of time you rest before beginning another exercise or another set of the same exercise. The repetition of a number of exercises without a break is called a set. For example: If I do an exercise and rest, then do the same exercise again, I have completed two sets. If I lifted one hundred pounds ten times and did that three different times, resting between each ten, that would be three sets of ten repetitions. Whenever you stop the exercise to rest, you have completed a set. A set could be just one repetition or it could be one hundred repetitions or more. Rest periods can vary significantly. My recommendation is to take sixty to ninety seconds to rest between each set. (Sixty seconds is preferable.)

6. **Exercises:** the specific activities included in a weight-resistance workout. This decision will be determined by available equipment, preference of equipment, and the specific body areas that you decide to exercise during a workout. I recommend exercises that involve the

main parts of the body, including the chest, shoulders, biceps, triceps, quadriceps, hamstrings, calves, back, and abdominal areas. You can either include an exercise for each body area in a workout or work certain body areas during one workout and other body areas on other workout days. I recommend alternating weight-resistance exercises between upper and lower body workouts. For example, you could focus on the upper body on Mondays (chest, shoulders, biceps, triceps, and back); lower body on Wednesdays (quadriceps, hamstrings, calves, and abdominals); and upper body again on Fridays. The following week you would begin Monday with lower body exercises again. This is an effective way to exercise the entire body and allow adequate rest and recovery for your muscles.

The Methods

No matter whether you have free weights or access to them, you can do weight-resistance exercises. This section discusses the three main methods.

Using Free Weights

For illustration purposes, I will assume that one has access to dumbbells and barbells. This may be equipment you have at home or at a gym where you are a member. Through trial and error, the amount of weight you should be lifting will become much clearer within a week or two. You may pick different days for your workout, but the goal is to set aside three days a week for the following workouts. Below is a chart for an upper body workout schedule for forty-five minutes or less. This first workout includes exercises for the chest, back, shoulders, biceps, and triceps.

Sample Workout

Monday (First Weekly Workout)

Target Area	Exercise	Reps (Repetitions)	Rest
Chest	Bench Press	3 Sets/12 Reps	1 min.
Chest	Chest Fly	1 Set/12 Reps	2 min.
Back	Upright Row	3 Sets/12 Reps	1 min.
Back	Bent-Over Row	1 Set/12 Reps	2 min.
Shoulders	Overhead Press	3 Sets/12 Reps	1 min.
Shoulders	Lateral Raise	1 Set/12 Reps	2 min.
Biceps	Dumbbell Curl	3 Sets/12 Reps	1 min.
Biceps	Hammer Curl	1 Set/12 Reps	2 min.
Triceps	Lying Dumbbell Extension	3 Sets/12 Reps	1 min.
Triceps	Triceps Kickback	1 Set/12 Reps	End of workout

On Wednesday, follow a similar format but concentrate on lower body exercises and abdominals.

Wednesday (Second Weekly Workout)

Target Area	Exercise	Reps (Repetitions)	Rest
Quadriceps	Squat	3 Sets/12 Reps	1 min.
Quadriceps	Lunge	1 Set/12 Reps	2 min.
Hamstrings	Stiff-Leg Dead Lift	3 Sets/12 Reps	1 min.
Hamstrings	Leg Curl	1 Set/12 Reps	2 min.
Calves	Toe Raises with Weights	3 Sets/12 Reps	1 min.
Calves	Toe Raises One Leg with Weights	1 Set/12 Reps	2 min.
Abdominals	Crunches	3 Sets/50 Reps	1 min.
Abdominals	Oblique Crunch	1 Set/50 Reps	End of workout

On Friday, repeat the upper body workout you did on Monday. It may be necessary to adjust the weights that you lifted Monday, increasing for some exercises or reducing for other exercises. The weights that you lift should reflect your ability to lift maximum weights with proper form. On Monday of the next week, repeat the lower body workout you completed the previous Wednesday. In other words, do weight-resistance workouts three days per week (you pick the alternate days), alternating between upper and lower body workouts.

When you have completed workout sets of twelve repetitions and the weight you are lifting becomes easier to lift, it is appropriate to gradually and continually increase the weight. Sensible increases should be made. The exercise should become challenging as you approach twelve repetitions. When it becomes too easy, it is time to increase the resistance. You should never aim to do the same exercise with the same weight indefinitely. As you get stronger, the weights that you began with will seem lighter. A weight is too light when you can do more repetitions than are required. When you are able to increase the repetitions beyond twelve, it is time to increase the resistance.

Remember: Your goal should be to make the workouts challenging. If they are not challenging, the weights are too light. However, lifting form should not be compromised to lift heavier weights. The exercises should always be completed with good form to assure proper strength development and decrease the chance of injury. At the beginning of a workout program, it is helpful to have someone familiar with weight-training exercises go over each exercise with you and demonstrate the proper way to complete it. There are videos on the Internet that demonstrate how to do a variety of exercises. In a gym setting, there are always staff members who can help you with exercise execution.

Using Resistance Bands

There are other weight-resistance exercises besides weight lifting. Some individuals do not have access to weight lifting equipment, so a second option might be utilizing exercise bands. Exercise bands can be purchased at a reasonable price and take up much less room than dumbbells or barbells. These exercise bands usually come in different colors that represent different levels of tension. It is more difficult to make measurable and incremental resistance increases with bands because they are not calibrated in pounds, as are dumbbells and barbells. There are three ways you can increase resistance with exercise bands: you can add additional bands, use stronger tension bands, or shorten a band by stepping on part of it or wrapping part of it around your hand. Using bands with greater tension has the same effect on your muscles as adding more weight with barbells or dumbbells. Exercise bands are typically used in rehabilitation settings to help individuals regain strength lost due to an accident, an injury, or a disability. When you purchase exercise bands, directions will be included, and there are videos on the Internet demonstrating how to perform band exercises. Both are good sources to learn how to complete your workout properly.

Using Your Body Weight

A third option is available for those who have no access to exercise equipment, a gym, or exercise bands. You can still complete some weight-resistance exercises by using your own body weight. Exercises such as abdominal crunches, push-ups, pull-ups, lunges, wall squats, yoga, and other exercises can make up your workout. This option is not the best one for every body area; however, push-ups and pull-ups are two of the very best upper body exercises. With some creativity, it is possible to develop a weight-resistance workout using only your body weight as resistance. The Internet has information regarding body-resistance exercises that would be appropriate for strength development.

Belonging to a gym will allow you to have access to barbells, dumbbells, and other weight-training equipment that is typically not available in the home. However, since not everyone has this option, resistance bands and home exercises offer good alternatives to a gym membership. This may be the necessary starting point for many. The focus should always be on what you *can* do rather than what you *cannot* do. Something is always better than nothing!

Stretching

The fourth basic exercise component is stretching. Stretching is important for increasing and preserving your flexibility. Stretching is essential in maintaining your body's range of motion.[8] As you age, your muscles tighten, and the range of motion within your joints tends to decrease. If you avoid stretching in your exercise routine you risk the possibility of losing your ability to complete daily activities. Lack of flexibility is now seen to be a major cause of general health problems and sports injuries. It is being linked to everything from stress, back pain, and even osteoarthritis. It also affects nagging injuries, especially around your joints, which take longer to heal. Some studies indicate that up to 60 percent of people with back and knee problems have tight hamstrings and hips. The main cause of these problems is a lack of flexibility.

You should focus on stretching these areas: neck, lower back, groin and hips, hamstrings, upper back, and shoulders. There are a number of videos on the Internet that illustrate different stretches as well as drawings that illustrate and explain how to complete the stretches. Yoga is a great form of exercise that builds strength, flexibility, and balance. It consists of a series of poses that can be tailored to virtually all body types, ages, and abilities. In many communities, there are classes offering yoga instruction.

Regardless of your age or your current level of flexibility, you can learn to stretch. Stretching does not require a huge time commitment and should be part of your daily routine. At the minimum, I recommend ten to fifteen minutes of stretching before beginning an exercise routine. Stretching prepares the muscles for activity because it increases blood flow and increases muscle temperature. Since muscles work best when they are warm, stretching helps to avoid injuries. The more flexible your muscles and tendons become, the better your body can handle the rigors of exercise and daily life activities. You should also include ten to fifteen minutes of stretching at the end of each workout because it aids in muscle recovery and eases soreness.

I will admit that for many years I did not take stretching as seriously as I should have. I did not realize how important stretching was to my overall physical well-being. Today I stretch for fifteen minutes before starting my workout, stretch during my workout between sets, and stretch after my workout. Consider these important potential health benefits of a regular stretching program:

- Preventing a loss in your range of motion
- Increasing the range of motion in your muscles
- Decreasing muscle tension throughout your body
- Increasing muscle strength
- Increasing muscle control

- Restoring muscle balance in your body
- Preventing injuries
- Increasing flexibility and range of motion in your joints
- Improving circulation
- Improving posture
- Increasing coordination and balance
- Relieving stress

When stretching you should follow the following guidelines:

1. Stretch slowly and comfortably.
2. Breathe naturally; do not hold your breath. Exhale during exertion, and inhale during relaxation.
3. Stretching should be a slow, sustained lengthening of the muscle. Do not bounce. Think "slow and deliberate."
4. Never stretch to the point of pain. If stretching becomes painful, you are stretching too far. Mild discomfort is acceptable.
5. Hold your stretches for between ten to thirty seconds.
6. You may repeat stretches two or three times.

In summary, a balanced exercise program that will maintain or increase your overall fitness level will consist of:

1. Three or four aerobic exercise workouts each week, with each workout lasting twenty to sixty minutes. For those who are unable to participate in aerobics, walking thirty to sixty minutes a day should be included in place of aerobics.
2. Walking an additional thirty minutes each day and completing a minimum of ten thousand steps each day.
3. Three weight-resistance workouts per week on alternate days of the aerobic workouts. Weight-resistance workouts should last between thirty to forty-five minutes each.

4. Light stretching for ten to fifteen minutes before and after each workout. See the sample workout schedule in the appendix.

With these balanced activities in your exercise program, you are prepared to raise and maintain the level of your personal health.

PART III:

FINDING AND MAINTAINING MOTIVATION

Chapter 9:

Setting Goals

We live in a society that often uses the word *busy* to explain our daily activities. Sometimes we get so "busy" doing certain things that we fail to take the time to do those things that should be done. It is easy to develop an imbalance with our time. We may spend far too much time on certain activities and far too little time on equally important issues. When you say that you are too busy for a responsibility, you may very well be saying that it is a low priority. It may be that you have poor planning and organization. Since you cannot increase the length of a day, it is important to periodically evaluate your priorities and evaluate where your time is being spent. Goal setting is an effective tool to clarify those things that you desire to accomplish and provide a timeline for their completion.

You may have been blessed with life experiences that nurture good and productive habits. It is highly likely, though, that you practice some habits that produce negative consequences. You can either cling to behavior that denies you the opportunity to accomplish what you would like to achieve or you can change and move in a different, more positive direction. You really only have two choices. You can stay the same, or you can change.

Habits are an accumulation of your present routines that you do automatically. Sometimes you may not even be aware of your habits because your brain allows you to perform your habits with little or no thought. You may have at least a general understanding of those things that you ought to do even though you are not presently doing them. Why? Since your present habits are on autopilot, you spend little time on planning how to change those habits that you know you should remove. To become effective in establishing new habits, it is essential that you understand that you must make planning a priority. Without planning, you will continue to engage in those habits that you have already established. This is certainly true when it comes to the decisions that you make each day concerning your health. Most of your health decisions are made automatically based on your present habits. These habits pertain to the foods that you eat, when you eat, the foods that you purchase at the grocery store, the amount of food that you eat each meal, and your level of physical activity each day. Your health today is directly related to the health habits that you practice on a regular basis. So the first step toward changing your health habits is evaluating your present habits.

Evaluating Your Habits

In order for you to understand why you have your present habits, you must evaluate your present routines. Each habit has a reason for existing. You need to ask yourself *why* you have the present habits that you do. Take a close look at each of the habits that you want to change and analyze why it exists. Your present habits must be doing something for you or you wouldn't be engaging in them. Your task is to determine whether your present habits are acceptable in light of the unhealthy consequences that they may be creating.

There are many unhealthy habits that people practice. Some habits result in sickness, debilitating diseases, or even death. It would be helpful for you to take the time to seriously evaluate your present habits to determine if you are doing some things that you really need or want to change. Some examples of unhealthy habits may include: consuming an excess of calories, eating too many saturated fats, eating too many trans fats, eating too many high glycemic carbohydrates, eating heavy meals in the evening, eating too many calories during any given meal, not drinking enough water, not getting enough fiber in your diet, not eating enough fruits and vegetables, overconsumption of alcohol, overconsumption of colas or other sugar-laden drinks, skipping breakfast, and relying on meals from fast food restaurants. The list could be longer, but these are some of the unhealthy choices that many people in America make. Some of these choices may be habits that you can use as goals to improve your personal health.

Begin by taking the time to specifically identify the new habit or habits that you desire to develop as a replacement for your present habits. It is important to have a strong enough reason to change habits. My experience is that unless you have a compelling reason to change, it is unlikely that a long-term change will occur. If it's "no big deal" then I expect no big change. Changing your habits will require some work on your part. When you decide to replace an undesirable habit for a desirable one, you need to understand how to do it. Planning is necessary. When I decided to begin an exercise program, I could only make the change if I got up earlier. To fit the routine into my day, I needed to begin my workout at 5:30 a.m. Without a strong reason to change, I could never have done it because I really didn't want to exercise that early in the morning. *But* my desire to change was stronger than my dislike of an early morning workout. This was an important mental decision that I made at the very beginning.

Starting new habits requires that you commit to a new plan. I had to make plans so that I could be down at the gym early each morning. I had to get to bed earlier than I was accustomed to. I had to set my alarm with the commitment to actually get out of bed and leave for the gym. Once you have decided to initiate a new habit, you need to create a habit-changing plan. To rid yourself of unhealthy habits, you need to create a plan for changing your habits.

Creating a Habit-Changing Plan

There are certain steps that you must take to change your undesirable habits. Change is difficult for almost everyone. It is simply easier and more comfortable to continue doing what you are used to doing. One definition of a habit is that it is "an automatic pattern of behavior to a specific situation." It may be inherited or acquired through frequent repetition. Remember that bad habits involving your thoughts, time, words, and actions have been acquired over weeks, months, and years. To be more concise—your habits are no accident! Whatever your current habits are, for better or worse, they simply *are*. This awareness can be an important reminder to you that if you truly want change, you'll need to do some things differently.

The definition of a good habit is one "that produces desirable results." When you become frustrated with your results or desire to achieve new results, you will then need to decide if you are willing to take new steps to acquire a new habit. If you decide not to change, the saying holds true, "If you do what you've always done, you will get what you've always gotten." You cannot get different results until you make the decision to engage in different habits. One way to change a bad habit is to follow these specific steps:

1. **Write down, specifically, what you would like to change or do and when you expect the results to happen.** Example: I want to lose five pounds within the next fourteen days. When you keep your plans for change exclusively in your mind, you can easily and often conveniently dismiss them as life events occur. Research proves that the act of writing down a goal is part of the mental process that helps you follow through. Because it is written, you can review it daily, which will help keep you focused and motivated. When you commit a plan to paper, you set a course. Keep it simple and focus on one habit change at a time. This is your best chance for success. Add to your successful changes as you create new habits. Various sources report that it takes between twenty-one and sixty-six days to develop a new habit. Rather than overwhelm yourself with too many changes, select one and plot your progress for a thirty-day period. You should make changes in incremental steps. For example, if you do not presently exercise, set a time at the beginning of ten to fifteen

minutes and continue this change for the next thirty days. If you can remain focused and consistent, you will develop a new habit.

2. **Identify the obstacles, challenges, and excuses that get in the way of change.** It is more effective to record your challenges before they occur so that you can develop a plan to overcome them. If you have failed to make desired changes in the past, analyze why you failed and consider what you can do to avoid future failures. For example, you may enjoy eating pizza in the evenings while you're watching TV because it relaxes you, or you may tend to skip meals early in the day because of your schedule and then consume most of your calories near the end of the day. Make plans for how you can overcome the obstacles and challenges that you identify. There will always be challenges with change. If you have a plan for how to react to those challenges, your likelihood of success will increase.

3. **Write down a specific plan to overcome each obstacle.** Examples: (1) I'll begin writing down what I eat in the evening, and I'll restrict myself to a healthy snack that is no more than three hundred calories. (2) I'll write down the number of calories that I eat in a day and restrict my total calories to no more than ten times my body weight or two thousand calories, whichever is less. (3) I'm going to eat a healthy breakfast each morning so that I can ignite my metabolism early in the day. (4) I'm going to pack healthy snacks and carry them with me so that I can have something healthy to eat every three hours. This will help distribute my calories over the day and ensure that I eat the majority of my calories before evening. All of these plans can help overcome potential obstacles that you may face during the day.

4. **List the benefits you hope to receive as a result of your change.** If you don't anticipate benefits, there will be no compelling reason to change. Example: I'm very

unhappy with my weight and I know that unless I make some changes I'm going to continue to be upset about it. I'll have a sense of accomplishment if I get my eating under control rather than allowing my busy schedule to dictate my eating habits. I know that I'll feel better physically and mentally if I can lose unhealthy weight, because it really bothers me. These are examples of benefits that you can look forward to realizing.

5. **Decide whether the benefits are worth the change to you.** You will need to decide if the change is something you really want or if it is just a good idea that you're not willing to put much effort toward achieving. If you decide that you really want to change, you must accept it as a commitment. You need to get focused and prepare your mind and spirit for the self-control and discipline required to undertake the task. If you cannot come to the conclusion that your stated goal is worth the change, it is unlikely that a change will actually happen. Your motivation to change is crucial if a change is going to occur.

As a follow-up to these five steps, leave visual reminders on your desk, refrigerator, or bathroom mirror to help you keep focused. Just talking about changing a habit and continuing with the same behavior as before will not result in a change.

Setting Goals

Setting effective goals is essential and requires thinking about what you really want to accomplish in your life. Goals provide you with targets at which you can aim. They help you to commit your time and effort and provide you with motivation. Most of all, goals provide a roadmap to take us from where we are to where we want to be. Yogi Berra's words on the subject are so true: "If you don't know where you're going, chances are you will end up somewhere else."

Your odds of success increase significantly when you make a decision to select a goal that you seriously and enthusiastically want to achieve. Setting goals based on your feelings at a given moment of time will make them more difficult to attain. Goals that are well thought out tend to bring about the most positive results. Anything that requires change also requires motivation. The greater your motivation, the more likely you are to succeed.

Many research studies have reinforced the power of writing down goals. One famous Harvard Business School study demonstrated that written goals could translate into earnings of ten times more money than those people who failed to establish goals and put them in writing. It was revealed in this thirty-year research study that only three percent of Harvard Business School graduates wrote down their goals. Of the remaining 97 percent, 11 percent had goals but failed to write them down, and 86 percent had not yet established goals at all. However, the three percent who had written down their goals were making ten times more income than the average of all other graduates. In addition, ninety-eight percent of the total wealth resided with that three percent who created written goals.[1]

Understanding the Value of Goals

Effective goal setting can be very helpful in making progress in almost all areas of life. Goals demand a focus and when you are focused, the likelihood of success will greatly increase. Goals can be very effective in these six major areas of life: (1) family and home, (2) spirituality and ethics, (3) social and cultural life, (4) finance and career, (5) physical health, and (6) mentality and education. Significant progress in these areas can be achieved through the development of weekly, monthly, quarterly, and annual goals. Goals are an important step in providing direction to your life. The extreme opposite of goal setting is aimlessly going through life with little or no planning, hoping that something might become different or get better. Proverbs 16:9 says, "A man's heart deviseth his way: but the Lord directeth his steps." If we fail to plan, we plan to fail!

Your Goals and Action Steps

There are a number of steps you can take to pinpoint which goals you truly want to achieve:

1. **Clarify your vision.** What is your primary objective? It is absolutely essential that you are working for something that you really want, not just something that sounds good. It is essential that you have a clear understanding of *why* you want to set the goal. If not, you will have trouble at the very beginning.

2. **Identify potential pitfalls.** Change does not come automatically. It requires a keen understanding of the obstacles, challenges, or limitations that may sabotage your efforts. You must identify these issues because change is always accompanied by challenge. Failure to identify obstacles will catch you off-guard and distract you. Remember this: "Every ceiling, when reached, becomes a floor upon which one walks." Embrace the challenges, stay focused, and remember that achievement is more of an endurance race than a sprint. Patience and perseverance are necessary qualities when pursuing any goal.

3. **Identify your goals for the next six months to a year.** Many people will likely tell you that you need to set realistic goals. There can be a problem with this advice. The opposite of this advice is "Shoot high to achieve high." You do not want to restrict yourself by setting goals that are not very challenging. For example, if you were one hundred pounds overweight and you began some new healthy eating habits, it would be unacceptable to set a goal to lose five pounds in a month. That would be an example of a goal that lacked a reasonable challenge. Most people who are at a healthy weight could easily lose five pounds in a month if that were their goal.

Setting low goals is not uncommon. Many people set goals that are way too low, and you need to be careful that you are not one of them. I believe that you need to set high goals and work toward them. You may actually accomplish more by setting high goals and not reaching them than you would by setting lower goals and achieving them. Self-limiting thoughts and behaviors can provide you with all of the reasons why you *can't* do something. But the Bible says that as Christians we are more than conquerors. Let's act like it! Sometimes you really do not understand how much you can achieve until you just go for it. For example, when our country first set a goal to put a man on the moon, many people thought it was an unrealistic goal. Though it was indeed challenging and ambitious, it was achieved. Therefore, my advice to you is to make your goals challenging yet attainable. Expect yourself to do your best!

Throughout history, every new useful invention may have been considered to be unrealistic (for example, telephone, Internet, and television). Wilbur Wright, one of the brothers given credit for the invention of the airplane, once said, "If we all worked on the assumption that what is accepted as true was really true, there would be little hope of advance." No great success began with the "good enough" mind-set. Change your mind and change your results!

4. **Based on your expectations, name three action steps that you need to take *today* to move closer to your goals.** Next, name three action steps that you need to take this week and then this month. Remember these words from Robert Collier: "Success is the sum of small efforts, repeated day in and day out."

Tip: Write your goals down and place them where you will see them *every* day. Goals not written down are only dreams. Although there is nothing wrong with dreams and good ideas that may come into your mind, the process of putting your goals down in writing is critical to directing your efforts toward actually achieving them.

Make Your Goals Meaningful

All strong goals have the same features and components. The following guidelines will enhance your efforts to develop effective, achievable goals:

1. **Start written goals with a verb because verbs are action words.** Examples: Walk a minimum of thirty minutes each day. Drink ten to twelve glasses of water each day. Eat a minimum of six servings of fruits and/ or vegetables each day.
2. **Avoid all goals that do not require personal responsibility.** "Get my wife to cook healthy meals" and "Work out with my neighbor three times per week" are two examples of goals that require *somebody else* to do something for the goal setter. The goal setter cannot do these things without someone else. An effective goal is one that you have the sole responsibility to complete and that does not depend upon the actions of others to be completed.
3. **Each goal should be measurable and have a timeline.** Each goal should have a deadline attached to it. Goals without deadlines lack the power of completion that they need to have. Examples: Lose five pounds in two weeks. Walk thirty minutes without stopping. Have at least a thirty-minute aerobic workout three days per week. You should always be able to evaluate your success regarding a goal by answering "Yes, I achieved it" or "No, I didn't achieve it."
4. **Make goals specific.** When you write effective goals that are clear, you will be able to determine whether the goal was or was not achieved. Vague goals are not measurable. Examples of vague goals, which you want to avoid, include: "I want to get closer to the Lord." "I want to help others." "I want to lose weight." "I want to get in shape." "I want to serve the Lord." Examples

of specific goals would be: "I'm going read my Bible for thirty minutes each day." "I will volunteer for two hours a week at the Senior Center." "I will lose three pounds within the next seven days." "I will volunteer to work in the church nursery one Sunday each month."

5. **Make sure your goals are achievable.** We would probably all agree that a goal to fly on our own volition like birds would be inappropriate because it is impossible for human beings to fly. The goal has to be achievable, not one that defies the principles of nature or of creation. You should be able to conclude either "Yes, I achieved it" or "No, I did not achieve it."

6. **Make sure your goals are challenging and require some effort.** Though goals should be possible to achieve, you need to be careful about setting your goals too low. Setting an achievable goal is not an excuse to set an achievable goal that is not challenging.

7. **Devise goals that are consistent with your values.** You should only set goals to achieve those things that you truly believe are worthwhile goals. Example: Read two chapters of a selected book in the Bible every day. This would be a goal consistent with the values of a Christian.

There are many reasons why people do not set goals even though they desire change in their life. I have identified five below:

1. **No compelling reason to set goals.** The stronger the reason you have for wanting to make a change and set a goal, the greater the likelihood of success. This is crucial to goal setting. When a strong reason to change is absent, goal achievement is diminished.

2. **Failure to realize the power and value of goal setting and achievement.** Just because you do not understand that there is an effective process for change does not alter the fact that one exists. This lack of awareness is

a stumbling block for those who do not understand the power of goal setting. Some people are willing to attribute the success of others to luck even when their achievement is directly proportional to the power of goal setting.

3. **Lack of awareness regarding how to set goals.** Many people haven't learned the mechanics of goal setting. People get wishes, dreams, and goals mixed up. They are not the same. A wish involves those things that you desire or want without having to commit to doing anything about it. A wish list is a list of everything that you may need or want someday but are not actively pursuing. Example: You may say, "I'd like to lose weight," but do nothing to make it happen. Dreams are the ultimate realization of your desires or wishes. They can be big and seem unrealistic at first. They are not as focused or specific as goals are, sometimes looking five, ten, even twenty years into the future. Dreams are your ultimate destination. Example: "My dream is to have a healthy and fit body that gives me energy and allows me to have a purposeful, enjoyable life." Goals are the intermediate steps that serve as stepping stones toward realizing your dreams. They are focused, specific, short-term, measurable targets that involve things under your direct control. Example: Walk a minimum of thirty minutes every day. That is one goal that may contribute to the dream of having a healthy and fit body.

4. **Fear of failure**. Most of us understand logically that we cannot achieve anything unless there is a change. However, many are afraid to take the steps necessary for change to occur because they fear that they will not accomplish what they set out to do and they believe that would make them appear to be failures. In all honesty, the ultimate failure is the failure to try. A failure to start or try is a guarantee that success is impossible. The counter-argument to the fear of failure is "What

do you have to lose?" Some people fear the rejection they may experience if they attempt something and fail to receive approval from others. Others are fearful because they just do not know what to expect; they fear the unknown. Some, even though they are not pleased with a particular situation, are more comfortable with the predictable. One of my favorite quotes is, "Do the things you fear the most, and fear will die a sudden death." This reminds me that most of our fears are mental figments, totally unfounded, with no concrete reason to believe they will actually become real and threatening. By being fearful, we guarantee that we will never accomplish what we really desire. Fear is an enormous enemy to progress!

5. **Feel they are too busy or disorganized.** Some people feel that change is just too much work and takes away from other things in life. It is true that setting and working toward goals takes time. It is also true that we all have the same amount of time in a day—24 hours to be exact. It is one of the few areas of life where there is true equality. The "I'm too busy" excuse may simply mean "This is a low priority and not worth my effort." All you can do is take one step at a time. One step at a time allows you to focus on the small pieces rather than on the finished work that may encompass many details. Identify the significant pieces that will help you achieve your final goal and proceed forward in a focused, methodical manner, one step at a time. Eventually, you will achieve your goal.

It is very important that you believe in the Lord—and yourself—to accomplish those things that you set out to achieve. Hebrews 11:6 reminds us, "But without faith it is impossible to please Him: for he that cometh to God must believe that He is, and that He is a rewarder of them that diligently seek Him." Luke 1:37 tells us, "For with God nothing shall be impossible." So if you have faith and you believe that God can accomplish anything, why would you be so easily dissuaded from believing that you can accomplish what you set out to do? God is not the problem!

Unfortunately, we human beings have learned to develop a number of excuses and self-limiting beliefs that undermine our belief in ourselves. Some common examples of self-limiting beliefs are "I'm too old," "I'm too young," "I'm too heavy," "I have a bad knee/hip/you name it," "I can't do it," "I'll make a fool out of myself," "I might do it wrong," "I might fail," "I'm not good enough," "I don't deserve it," "It's not a spiritual issue," "I'm not important enough," "I'm too busy," "My wife doesn't support me," "My husband doesn't support me," "Other people will laugh at me," "This problem runs in my family—I can't help it," "I have other conflicts," and "I'm not smart enough." Self-limiting thoughts can actually paralyze you from taking any meaningful action toward accomplishing a goal. Thoughts are not necessarily a true reflection of reality and often are nothing more than lies. Most of the time, "Change your mind, change your results" is a rallying cry to overcome self-limiting behaviors. Your thoughts must shift *first*, and then your thoughts must be followed up by action that leads to change.

It is important for you to take an inventory of your life from time to time. Where are you today? What is it that you would like to change or that you need to change? If there are things that should be done to change the course of your life, following the goal setting guidelines in this chapter is an effective process that can bring direction, focus, and the completion of those things that are presently only wishes or dreams! Philippians 3:14 says, "I press toward the mark for the prize of the high calling of God in Christ Jesus." It is the completion of your goals that allows you to reach your desired outcome and your potential! Get started and set the goals that you long to achieve. Today is the day!

Chapter 10:

What's Eating You?

Many Americans live in fast-paced environments with many expectations and responsibilities that, if not contained, could overwhelm anyone. These everyday situations have the potential to create stress, disappointment, discouragement, and feelings of failure. If not addressed, these situations create internal emotional turmoil. One way some deal with this emotional turmoil is by medicating themselves with food. Food has become some people's drug of choice. The improper use of food can be compared to alcohol abuse, drug abuse, and other unhealthy behaviors that keep some of us from being the people that God wants us to be. It is very important to periodically take an inventory to determine whether something is causing you emotional distress. If so, problems can either be ignored or addressed. Addressing problems and issues by pursuing healthy solutions is the desirable course of action. So, what's eating you?

Sometimes having the information you need to control your weight is just not enough to get results. Many people struggle to stay on a healthy diet despite their best intentions. They want to lose weight, but they can't say no to the unhealthy foods they enjoy most. Restrictive diets can be especially challenging for people who have emotional eating problems. Food has become a comforter for many people, and any threat to or attempt to restrict the food of an emotional eater can be disastrous. In addition, some people eat when stressed, lonely, or anxious. This is fairly common, and it does not mean you have a serious problem. Just recognizing that fact and planning a strategy to deal with it may be all that is required to overcome these eating problems.

This chapter will not be relevant to everyone who reads it, but surely almost everyone will be able to identify with emotional eating. A word of caution: this discussion is not meant to cause people to become overly involved in introspection and seek a reason for lack of success in losing weight. It should instead motivate you to ask some questions to see if there is a possible link between your emotions and what you eat.

The Bible tells us that the Spirit is willing but the flesh is weak. Each of us must realize that before we can solve a problem, it is important to first understand what the problem is. It is only natural to think about your problem of overeating and wonder what is causing it. Some people have experienced repeated failures with losing weight. There are many reasons for this. Failure may be due to a lack of self-control, commitment, focus, or knowledge. While in many cases these may appear to be the reasons why you are not successful in losing weight, your emotional state is the real root cause.

In this chapter, you will find questions that you should ask yourself to see if there is a connection for you between food and emotions. If you answer yes (or "possibly yes") to these questions, you may better understand and identify the obstacles that you need to overcome. Others may realize after reading this chapter that their eating problems are more severe than normal. Those individuals may want to seek additional insight through other literature or by obtaining professional help.

There is a vast amount of information regarding what foods to eat, what portions to eat, the number of calories to eat, and other guidelines for healthy nutritional eating. This is all good information to seek out if you lack this knowledge; however, there may be hidden emotional reasons which undermine your success. Knowing what to eat and how much to eat will have little impact on your success unless emotional issues are addressed first. This chapter provides you with information to help you understand if emotional issues are obstacles in obtaining your healthy body weight. If this is the case, I have outlined some practical strategies that may help you overcome the emotional issues that are presently sabotaging your success.

Eating problems are described as an addiction, a disorder, a compulsion, or as emotional eating. Professionals disagree on what exact term is applicable. For our purposes, we will refer to eating problems as emotional eating because it describes a problem that is emotionally based. Anorexia and bulimia will not be discussed except to say that professional help is often required to overcome these disorders. It is important to understand that some people are truly addicted to food just like others are addicted to alcohol, cigarettes, or drugs. They simply cannot, no matter how hard they try, end the addiction without additional, professional help.

A Close Look at Emotional Eating

So, what is emotional eating? Emotional eating is the practice of consuming large quantities of food—usually comfort food—in response to feelings instead of in response to hunger. Emotional eating is eating for any reason other than nutrition. The goal of an emotional eater is to derive some sort of comfort from eating and to find a way to cope with the situations that they are confronted with on a day-to-day basis. Emotional eating is a prevalent habit and a part of our culture. People use food to celebrate, to deal with unpleasant feelings, to cope with problems at work or conflicts, to combat boredom, and for many other reasons unrelated to proper nutrition. Emotional eating is not recognized as a significant problem in our society, but since two-thirds of all Americans are either overweight or obese, I think it is safe to say that it is indeed a significant problem.[1] When compared to many well-publicized addictions in our society, emotional eating and overeating are minimized!

Who could be considered an emotional eater? An emotional eater is a person who eats to satisfy emotional issues in his or her life. These people may or may not be aware of their emotional connection to food. These individuals may be overweight by as little as a few pounds—or as much as a few hundred pounds. They are drawn to food just like an alcoholic is drawn to alcohol or in the way a workaholic gravitates toward work. They have a strong emotional reliance on something on the outside to make them feel good on the inside. Emotional eaters consume food to fill a void.[2]

In order to facilitate good emotional health, people need to have their physical and emotional needs met. Some of these emotional needs are for feelings of security, control, achievement, and purpose. People also need friendship, intimacy, and emotional connection to others. The failure to have these needs met, whether intentional or unintentional, creates potential problems. Emotional eating can be the response to unmet emotional needs. Emotional eating can be triggered by a number of factors related to unmet needs created by such things as a dysfunctional family, a setback in life, a disappointing marriage, a job failure, a death in the family, or a serious illness. These situations can lead to emotional deficits that can trigger negative responses. Emotional eating is but one way to respond negatively.

It is important, when dealing with emotional eating, to stop denying that it is a problem. Denial makes it impossible to solve an eating problem. Even when you understand that you have an eating problem, you may not understand the depth of it. Sometimes it is difficult to see yourself as you are, because denial may not allow you to see your emotional dependence on food objectively. Developing an awareness of this truth is the key to breaking through denial. Without an awareness that you are in denial and the knowledge of how to overcome it, you may be vulnerable to more serious eating disorders that can be more difficult to overcome. Negative emotions such as low self-esteem, guilt, shame, anger, self-hatred, and feelings of being unloved can become more intense when emotional eating is not adequately addressed.

There are many reasons why people overeat. Consider these common reasons for emotional eating:

1. **Cultural pressures.** There is an overwhelming amount of advertising urging people to eat. Television ads and

an overabundance of fast food restaurants advertise high-calorie, high-fat meals for just a few dollars. Food is so readily available that Americans have gone from eating one meal outside the home each month to eating an average of one outside meal per day. The continuous signals that you see and hear each day can trigger a desire to eat. Advertising works! This massive amount of advertising has led us to be a food-obsessed society. It has caused Americans to become the most obesity-plagued society in the world.

2. **Love and intimacy.** Some people subconsciously desire to gain weight. This may occur after a traumatic event, such as a broken relationship. Food may be used as a tool to make yourself less attractive to others and deny your sexuality in order to avoid intimacy.

3. **Immediate gratification.** Some people turn to food as a form of self-managed gratification. Instead of building relationships or developing interests, food may fill this void. People pleasers who help in hospitals, schools, and churches may binge in private.

4. **Food as a tranquilizer.** Anxiety can create the desire to eat. Each time you eat, the brain stimulates neurological chemicals called endorphins, which are natural painkillers, relaxants, and pleasure stimulators. Endorphins can produce feelings similar to those generated by narcotic drugs. A true food addict reacts in a similar manner as a drug addict.

5. **Avoiding problems.** When you get into the habit of not dealing with issues in your life, it becomes easy to turn to food as a means of escape.

6. **Punishing yourself or others.** When you are angry about something you have done, it can create a sense of guilt. One way that you can punish yourself is by overeating and gaining weight. Your weight gain then becomes your reason to punish yourself. This may be less painful than dealing with the anger that was created

by your initial guilt. You can become obese not only to punish yourself, but also to use weight as a scapegoat. Saying, for example, "I don't deserve to look pretty." Or you could so twist your thinking that you could believe that "If I just stay fat and unhappy for the next ten years, then I've paid the debt for my guilt." Some people gain weight to punish their spouses in relationships they have come to view as mistakes.

7. **Relieving depression or stress.** This can be the result of repressed anger or an unconscious desire to get vengeance on someone. When you hold a grudge it becomes an emotional, spiritual, and physical problem. When you hold resentment against God or others, the resentment causes serotonin and epinephrine to be depleted in your brain cells. As a result, you lose energy and motivation. Depletion of brain chemicals can cause you to gain weight because of inactivity. In those who have repressed anger, there is both a chemical and emotional basis for overeating. Many people literally repress their anger by putting food on top of it. This hostility may originate from a person's childhood or from current situations.

8. **Rebelling against oneself or others.** You may overeat out of frustration over trying to live up to the "perfect" body images that are prevalent in advertising. This frustration can be directed toward parents, a spouse, or others.

9. **Need for control.** The oldest child is often overly controlled by new parents, and this first child may be anxious to do a good job. Fifteen of the first sixteen astronauts were the first-born children in their families. Perfectionists can become a great asset to themselves and society, but this tendency can also lead to compulsive eating. Control can become a major issue for children growing up in a dysfunctional family. When there is abuse in a family, children experience fear. In order to

survive and protect themselves from pain, they may desire to take more control of their life. Many emotional eaters have been excessively disciplined.

10. **Faulty perception of body image.** It is possible to have a distorted self-image. You may lose interest in your body image as your emotional eating becomes more frequent or more serious. This faulty perception can lead to denial and an inability for you to see the truth regarding your dependence upon emotional eating.

11. **Emotional feelings about food developed in one's family.** Patterns of behavior experienced at mealtimes during childhood may have an emotional impact on a person's present eating habits. This impact may have been affected by past behaviors such as whether overeating was a typical behavior at home, whether food was used to satisfy emotional issues in the home, how often food was used for celebrations, or if there was abuse in the family. When the dinner table is a battleground, tensions are created. Eating to celebrate can become a daily ritual. One may overeat to please parents and show that meals are enjoyed. One can also overeat to defy parents. These ingrained attitudes toward food can be factors in overeating.

12. **Attempting to satisfy a vacuum in one's life.** Food can be used to compensate for literally anything that has created a void in a person's life.[3]

Assessing Your Eating Patterns

It is important for you to become aware of your present eating patterns. This is especially true if you are a person whose eating is consistently stimulated by your emotional state. When you learn to identify your patterns of emotional eating and the feelings and circumstances that trigger it, you can then learn to experience your feelings without having to turn to food. This puts you in a position to solve problems by dealing with them at their source.

Ask yourself the questions below about your present eating habits. Answer them as honestly as you can. Your answers may reveal some evidence about whether or not you are an emotional eater. You may be an emotional eater if you answer yes to any of the following questions:

1. Do you ever eat without even realizing you're eating?
2. Do you often feel guilty or ashamed after eating?
3. After an unpleasant experience, do you eat even if you aren't feeling hungry?
4. Is your weight more than 20 percent higher than your ideal body mass index weight?
5. Do you crave certain foods when you're upset or depressed?
6. Have significant people in your life expressed concern about your eating patterns or your weight?
7. Do you always eat when you are happy?
8. Do you always eat when you are sad?
9. Do you feel the urge to eat after seeing food advertisements?
10. Do you eat because you do not seem to have anything else to do?
11. Does eating make you feel better when you're down?
12. When you're worried about something, does eating help you escape your worries?
13. Has your weight fluctuated by more than ten pounds in the past six months?
14. Do you often eat alone or in odd locations?
15. Do you always eat when you are bored?
16. Do you eat when you're angry?
17. Do you fear that your eating is out of control?
18. Do you hide food for yourself?
19. Do you always eat when you are anxious or nervous?
20. Are you embarrassed about your physical appearance?

The above questions are not intended to label you as an emotional eater. Instead, your answers may provide you with a greater understanding regarding the extent to which your emotions affect your eating.

Putting an End to Emotional Eating

Whenever you spend too much time numbing the pain of your emotions, you lose the capacity to deal appropriately with your problems. The fact that food has addictive properties that can also impact your mood will further complicate the situation. You may teach yourself that when you have a problem, the best way to solve it is by eating. Practiced enough, this can become a way of dealing with problems, and this habit can be difficult to break. This is the worst part about emotional eating. It actually causes your problems to multiply. It is a vicious cycle that keeps repeating itself until the cycle is broken.

Unless you learn how to stop emotional eating it will be impossible to lose weight and keep it off. It will be emotionally difficult to continue fighting this same internal battle. This battle will result in the loss of your personal joy.

In addressing any challenge, it is helpful to understand the nature of the problem. There are several things that may help you when trying to address this particular problem. Consider these steps to help you put an end to emotional eating:

1. Develop a different mind-set regarding food. The emotional eater tends to link food to pleasure. What I did when I made my lifestyle change was begin to see food as a source of energy to complete daily activities. I began to see food as a nutritional necessity. When I developed this mind-set I began to look at food as a means to an end—proper nutrition and a healthy body. For my body to operate efficiently I needed certain nutrients. This caused me to focus on whether my food choices fit my nutritional purpose or not. If a food had

a nutritional purpose, I included it in my diet. If a food did not have a positive nutritional purpose, I rejected it. This evolved into an "eating to live" mentality instead of a "living to eat" perspective. Eating is not a sport. Food sustains life and affects how well your body operates. When you begin to see and value whether food makes a positive contribution or a negative contribution, you begin to view food differently than just something used for convenience or for pleasure. This is an important change in your mental focus and moves you away from emotional eating behavior.

2. While making the transition to a new mind-set change, you will need to respond to cravings that you may experience. Keeping a journal to record your eating behavior will make it clear to you what emotions trigger your cravings and what types of foods you resort to when those cravings occur. When cravings do occur, you need to have a plan in place that will distract you so that you do not submit to the cravings. Cravings need to be suppressed for just a few minutes before they pass. If you have a plan to respond to these cravings before they occur, you are more likely to have success. For example you may develop a plan to take a ten to fifteen minute walk as soon as cravings occur.

3. You need to identify your hunger patterns so that you can put your distraction plan into action. The first distinction that you need to make is between real hunger and emotional hunger. The way I addressed this problem was by meal planning and scheduling definite eating times.

4. Plan your meals in advance. Do not leave eating to chance. It is too dangerous! When I decided to begin eating a healthy diet, I made a detailed plan. I planned to have a meal every two and a half to three and a half hours. I knew that I was going to have specific servings of food. One serving was going to be a healthy protein,

one serving was going to be a healthy carbohydrate, and the final serving was going to be either another healthy carbohydrate or a healthy fat. By organizing a plan with this structure, I limited my opportunity for emotional eating. This structured plan allowed me to lose forty pounds in twelve weeks and achieve a healthy body weight. Remember, when you fail to plan, you plan to fail!

5. The critical step in planning your meals in advance begins before you arrive at the grocery store. Make sure when you go to the grocery store that you are not hungry. It is imperative that if you plan to eat healthy you need to have healthy foods available at meal times. If you are like most people, you will eat any comfort food that you bring into your house. Don't buy those foods that tempt you to engage in emotional eating. You cannot eat foods that are not available. The groceries that you purchase should be those foods that you plan to eat each day for your meals. If you really want to make healthy changes, making healthy food choices is a priority and a necessity!

If you practice these steps, you will be taking some very important steps toward putting an end to emotional eating. I have personally applied them, so I know that they work. Do not be tempted to wing it when it comes to planning. More often than not, planning is the difference between success and failure!

Recognizing and Managing Your Triggers

Some foods seem to have a greater influence on emotional eating than others. The most common trigger foods in emotional eating are typically so-called comfort foods that are high in calories and low in nutritional value. This type of food often replaces the foods in your diet that your body needs to be healthy. High glycemic comfort foods often contribute to overeating. Sugar and chocolate are common food triggers. A sugar/fat combination is the most common trigger because it has especially potent mood-altering properties.[4] This combination medicates depression and boredom. It supplies a short-lived surge of energy because your body rapidly metabolizes glucose. But your body then demands even more sugar. Sugar is an "upper" and can also be a sedative. For example, table sugar is half glucose and half fructose. Glucose is absorbed in the blood stream extremely quickly, while fructose enters the blood stream at a slower, more controlled rate. Scientific evidence shows that the more sugar you eat, the more you want.

Chocolate is loaded with phenyl ethylamine, a chemical related to amphetamines. It raises blood pressure and blood glucose levels. After consuming phenyl ethylamine we feel more alert and have a feeling of well-being and contentment. It is believed to work by causing the brain to release b-endorphin, an opioid peptide, which is the driving force behind the pleasurable effects. It has been referred to as the "love drug." One way to decrease chocolate cravings is to take magnesium supplements. Since many Americans are deficient in magnesium, chocolate is often their source of this important mineral.[5] After foods containing sugar and chocolate, salty foods—like French fries and potato chips—are the next most common trigger food.

In addition to food triggers, you need to be aware that environmental factors and certain events are also effective triggers that can encourage emotional eating. This could include family gatherings, parties or banquets; experiencing peer pressure; encountering comfort foods at work, potlucks at church, or smorgasbords; driving past a fast food restaurant; seeing television ads; smelling foods; or grocery shopping.

Before you can mount a successful plan to eliminate your tendency to engage in emotional eating, you must first be able to recognize those events, emotions, or circumstances that trigger emotional eating. When you are able to develop a clear picture regarding the cause of these triggers you can then develop a plan to neutralize them. Every emotional eater has a unique personality and is in an environment with unique circumstances. It is therefore important to focus directly upon your own specific situation. Consider following these steps to gain a better understanding of the triggers that cause you to engage in emotional eating.

1. One effective way to identify your triggers is to keep a journal. You should write down every food you eat in a day. This should include all snacks and meals. You should also identify your emotions when you eat and write them down too. In addition to writing down when you eat, note any unique circumstances that occur prior to your eating. Focus on the details that are relative to the times that you eat. Did your eating have anything to do with the people who were around you? Was it your regular mealtime? Were you discouraged about anything? Did someone say something to you that hurt your feelings? Were you celebrating something? Were you lonely when you were eating? The answers to questions like these will help you better understand when and why your emotional eating occurs. For your journal to be effective in uncovering your emotional triggers, you will need to be very specific regarding details surrounding the time at which you decided to eat. Though the journal entries may seem cumbersome for you, remember that this is an important step so that you can develop a plan to rid your dependence on emotional eating. Keep this journal as long as it takes for you to see a definite pattern emerge. Though it may take longer, usually two to four weeks will be adequate. Remember, the more specific you are with details, the more meaningful your journal information will be.

2. Now that you have recorded your eating and emotional state in your journal, you are now ready to analyze your journal entries. As you review your journal, you should be able to see that there are certain patterns to your eating. You need to begin to look for common links in your eating patterns. For example, you may discover

that you engage in emotional eating when you are around your friends or acquaintances, or you may find that you tend to eat comfort foods more often when you are alone and feeling lonely. Look for links that answer the five *W*'s—*who* caused it, *what* circumstances caused it, *when* it was caused, *where* it was caused and *why* you believe it happened. The answers to these questions will help to clarify what triggers lead to your emotional eating.

3. Now that you more fully understand your triggers, you are now in a position to develop a plan to manage your triggers and combat the causes of your emotional eating. For additional strategies to overcome emotional eating, review the section below, "Planning Ahead for Success."

Planning Ahead for Success

Now that you are aware of the situations and circumstances that are responsible for creating the triggers that encourage your emotional eating, it is time to put a plan in place so that you can shed your reliance upon using food for emotional reasons. Knowing what to do is never enough—you must take action to get the results that you desire. Consider the following plans that can allow you to move forward with healthier eating:

1. Plan when you are going to eat. When you attach a time to when you eat, you have eliminated the option of eating based solely on your feelings. I recommend eating smaller meals every two and a half to three and a half hours.

2. Plan what you are going to eat before eating. Plans are essential to a healthy diet. Without a plan, you become vulnerable to eating based upon your emotions or circumstances. I recommend eating five or six smaller meals each day. Three meals should include: one

serving of a healthy protein, one serving of a healthy carbohydrate (fruit or vegetable), and one more serving of either another healthy carbohydrate or a serving of a healthy fat. The two or three additional meals or snacks should include only two servings. You can select your servings from these three choices: a healthy protein serving, a healthy carbohydrate serving, or a healthy fat serving. When you plan your meals ahead of time, you take your emotions out of the equation.

3. Eliminate the comfort foods that you have relied upon from your home. There is no logical reason why you should tempt yourself with foods that have been part of your past problems. If you do not purchase these foods, you remove your temptation.

4. Develop a plan for each of the emotional triggers that you have identified in your journal. These plans should be developed before you are confronted with the emotional temptations to eat as you have in the past. For example, you may have learned from your journal that you engage in emotional eating when you are lonely. You need to have a plan to counteract your loneliness with a new behavior. An example of your plan may be that when you feel lonely, you plan to take a fifteen-minute walk or call a friend on the telephone. Always create an alternative activity that you are willing and able to follow through with when emotional triggers impact you. The alternative activities will be unique to each of you. For the above example taking a fifteen-minute walk may or may not fit. Regardless, your task is to identify an alternative action that *will* fit you.

The key is to plan ahead. Put these plans in writing and review them so that you will be ready to implement new behaviors when negative emotions tempt you to engage in emotional eating. This process may seem unnatural to you at first but as you practice your plans

over a period of time, they will become your new habits
and will replace your emotional eating.

Do not minimize the importance of planning when making habit
changes in your life. Your present habits occur almost automatically,
with little thought. The only way to change these ingrained behaviors
is to develop new habits. Initially, these new habits must be carefully
planned. When you practice these new habits over time, they become
your new habits. This is exactly the end result that you are working
to accomplish—to replace the emotional eating habit with a new
habit that is healthier for you! Instead of wondering "What's eating
you?" aim to get to the place where your answer is "*Nothing* is eating
me!" Philippians 4:11 says, "Not that I speak in respect of want: for I
have learned, in whatsoever state I am, therewith to be content."

In theory, change is fairly easy in that many others have
accomplished the actions that you need to take. But we all tend to
get comfortable with the way that we do things. Our habits become
familiar to us, and we repeat them continuously with no conscious
thought. There are times when each of us realizes that a change
needs to be made. We realize that we are not going down the road
that God, in His perfect will for our life, would want us to go. This
is the time that we need to embrace change because of the positive
benefits that we can experience. You need to change your mind-set
and plan to take some intentional actions. Then and only then can
change take place. Just the knowledge of what to do will not cause
change to occur. Intentional actions must follow knowledge.

I have formulated twelve Healthy Vessels principles that may
just help you to make some of the mind-set changes that you need
to make. Read the twelve principles in the next chapter and make a
commitment to implement them as you make the lifestyle changes
necessary to improve your personal health.

Chapter 11:

Sticking to the Healthy Vessels Principles

In your quest to obtain optimal health, my hope and prayer is that you will be able to honestly utter the same words as Paul in 2 Timothy 4:7: "I have fought a good fight, I have finished my course, I have kept the faith." There is no doubt that you have the capacity to do what you need to do to change the habits that you need to change, because there is a source of strength that is available to you as a Christian. Philippians 4:13 reads, "I can do all things through Christ which strengtheneth me." Changing unhealthy habits is just one of those things! Consider the following principles and the mind-sets that may provide assistance to you while making positive health changes in your life.

1. **Your decision to change is your most important decision.**
    A decision is the act of making a judgment or making up your mind. A decision is not "wishy-washy." It does not fluctuate back and forth. It is an internal determination. A decision to change is most effective when you have decided that there is no turning back until you reach the desired outcome—regardless of the obstacles that may confront you. A proper mind-set is critical to

making any change. God has equipped you well to make the positive changes that you desire and need to make. When you make a decision, there is a new focus, and this new focus provides a greater motivation to do what is needed to attain the desired results. It is the foundation for change.

Decisions are typically made because of a desire to realize a stated concrete result, go in a new direction, reach a specific goal, or remove a certain condition or set of circumstances. Therefore, the reason "why" becomes very important. Without a strong reason, it is unlikely that you will expend or sustain the energy needed to make a meaningful change. Your decision to change is your *most* important decision.

2. **It's not where you start that matters—it's where you finish.**
Anytime you initiate a change, there is a set of steps or actions that must first be completed in order to achieve the desired result. This process can be discouraging to you if you expect results instantly or with a minimal amount of effort or change. The proper mind-set will require you to take the specific, step-by-step actions necessary to accomplish your goal. The process can be enjoyable and satisfying. It is important to enjoy the successes along the way by focusing on the progress that you are making rather than focusing on the fact that you are not there yet. Change requires effort, time, and patience. Satan will provide some resistance anytime you begin to make positive changes. Do not become impatient with how far you have to go. Instead, identify smaller incremental steps. Work toward those steps and celebrate your achievements along the way. Each step that you reach brings you that much closer to your final goal.

3. **Honoring God doesn't require that you've done the best—just that you've done *your* best.**

   Whether you succeed or not, God has blessed you with certain abilities and skills. Your challenge for any given task is to do your best, and that will be good enough. The only time you need to adjust your efforts is when you proceed in such a way that is not the best you can do. This requires an honest self-evaluation. You need to make sure that during this evaluation, you do not quit when faced with the challenges that are likely to occur. Obstacles and difficulties are to be expected when changes are pursued. Quitting when you are confronted with these roadblocks is not doing your best. Like it or not, you are in a battle with your flesh in this world. You should not exaggerate your efforts, nor should you engage in self-criticism regarding them. When you do the best you can do, that is all you can do.

4. **When faced with a challenge, look for a way—not a way out. Eliminate your excuses!**

   Some tasks are challenging and require special effort. *Effort* is not another word for impossible. You need to be sure, that in the quest to do your best, you are not sabotaging yourself by making excuses that prevent you from doing your best. There is some truth to the saying, "When the going gets tough, the tough get going." When confronted with difficulties, it is human nature to make excuses and rationalize why something cannot be done. This is especially true when you pursue endeavors outside of your comfort zone.

   Nearly all things in life that require change are neither simple nor easy. Those things that require special effort and perseverance have the potential to bring about the greatest personal satisfaction. This principle requires you to search yourself to determine how to overcome the obstacles that may stand in your way. Be slow to quit and quick to accept the challenges and obstacles that come your way. Quitting is taking the easy way out, and it gets much easier to quit the second time when you are challenged. Some of the greatest achievements made by man were not easy. Some of them actually seemed impossible to achieve—but they were not.

5. **Goals that are clearly defined and measurable are more likely to be accomplished.**
    It is always more likely that you will accomplish a goal when you have taken the time to specifically identify what the goal is. Undefined goals are really just wishes and dreams. When goals are vague and hazy, there is a greater chance for failure. When goals are clearly defined, it will be obvious if the goal has been achieved. You will be able to answer "Was the goal achieved?" with a yes or no answer. Not only should a goal be clearly defined, there should be a timeline attached to it. Failure to do so will allow for procrastination. When you fail to assign a specific deadline to achieve a goal, you increase the likelihood that the goal will not be achieved. Goals are really dreams with a timeline attached.

6. **Your biggest obstacle to good health may be your present habits.**
    When it comes to health habits in our society, you may often get caught playing "follow the leader." You may reason that since so many people eat meals at fast food restaurants, it can't be that bad. The medical evidence shows that we are becoming unhealthier as a nation. The surgeon general of the United States has announced publicly that obesity is the number one problem in America. That is quite a mandate when you consider all of the problems that we have in America today. When bad habits are practiced so widely, it is easy to embrace

them and make them your own personal habits. But sometimes it is wise to be different from the masses.

As Christians, we are to be the "light of the world." We cannot expect to duplicate unhealthy practices and be immune to the consequences. Since it takes some time before bad habits reveal undesirable results, you can easily become lulled to sleep, so to speak, and not realize the future dangers that you are creating for yourself. It is important that you take an inventory of some of your eating habits and evaluate whether they are habits that will create the long-term results that you desire. You can be your own worst enemy when it comes to your health. Free will and choice offer two options: make positive choices or negative ones. You need to ask yourself questions about your personal eating habits and whether you are eating in a manner that will promote optimum health. Are you already beginning to show symptoms of an unhealthy lifestyle? You need to ask yourself how well your personal choices are working for you. When you find areas that are not conducive to good health, you can either turn away from them and develop new habits or accept the risk factors that come with unhealthy choices.

7. **There are no shortcuts.**
In order to accomplish the things that you desire to do, you need a plan, and you must put forth some effort to execute the plan. We live in an age and culture that continually sends advertising messages that lead us to believe that we can get good health results with little or no effort. Magic pills, magic exercises, and other gimmicks are used to sell products. We are told that we can achieve good health by eating anything we want. We have been told almost every conceivable lie to entice us to buy products that promise instant results. These claims are just not true. There are some distinct

differences between healthy and unhealthy habits. In order for you to achieve good health it becomes necessary for you to follow sound nutritional guidelines. These guidelines will require some focus, discipline, and self-control. These are the qualities that advertising does not talk about very often. It may be appealing to believe that you can achieve your goals with little or no effort, but the evidence is just the opposite. Eating foods that are high in trans fats, saturated fats, and sodium and lacking in nutritional value is not healthy eating. Maintaining a sedentary lifestyle with little movement is also not healthy. Become informed, evaluate what you are presently doing, and make a decision to incorporate healthy practices that will really work for your benefit.

8. **Knowing is not enough—you must take action.**
Accomplishing anything in life always has some action attached to it. It is true that you need to know *what* to do before you can do it. This is the reason why knowledge is so important. Many people either do not know what to do or they make conscious decisions to practice unhealthy habits. Knowledge is very important, but when you fail to act upon knowledge, you will most likely get the same results as someone who lacks knowledge. The Bible is full of examples of people who knew what to do but failed to do it. Find out what you need to do and then take the actions that will lead to the accomplishment of your goals. The key to successful achievement is taking action by applying the knowledge that you have.

9. **In order to get what you desire, model someone who has already achieved it.**
This is a common-sense approach to learning how to do anything. If you want to become physically fit, would you follow the recommended advice of someone who is

physically fit or the advice of someone who has never been fit? If your goal were to stop smoking cigarettes, would you seek advice from someone who cannot stop or would you seek advice from those who have actually been able to break the habit? Those who have "been there and done that" are in a very unique position to help others conquer similar challenges. The best way to understand how to do almost anything is to find someone who has done it and find out how they did it. Success always leaves clues. Modeling is a faster way to success than trial and error.

10. **Success is the sum of small efforts, repeated day in and day out.**
Rome wasn't built in a day. Success takes time. For instance, if you are fifty pounds overweight, you are not going to lose that weight in a short time. Your success will come by making small changes every day to support your goal. You will reduce caloric intake, substitute healthy foods for the unhealthy ones that you were eating, follow the rules of good portion control, drink adequate amounts of water each day, and begin to increase movement by making intentional exercise a part of your lifestyle. Over time, you will be able to meet your goal of losing the fifty pounds. Never underestimate the importance of the small steps that are necessary for you to take in order to achieve a great result. A person with a focused mind who does the small things with consistency and persistence is the person who is most likely to succeed. The road to success is more like an endurance race than a sprint. Breaking goals down into small steps is a key strategy that leads to success. Remember, the tortoise always wins!

11. **A lifestyle change lasts a lifetime--not twelve weeks.**

Yo-yo diets are short-term activities. They may produce results; but when your old habits return, the temporary results will be wiped away. Statistics tell us that more than 95 percent of all diets fail. This is because they are temporary and unsustainable over time. You will only get results as long as you can sustain the behaviors or actions that caused you to get the results in the first place. A lifestyle change involves developing sound habits that are healthy and sustainable throughout your life. If your ideal weight was 130 pounds when you were twenty-five years of age, it is an ideal weight at ages thirty-five, forty-five and sixty-five. The key is to develop lifelong habits that support a healthy body. The diet plan of a typical American works well for book deals, but not for your long-term health. The principles introduced in Healthy Vessels are not just good practices for the twelve-week program. They are good, healthy habits that should be incorporated into all areas of your life and followed throughout your life.

12. **Your success grows when you pass your success on to others.**
    There are many people in our society who are in need of help with their health. Some people do not know what to do, and others need moral support. Some need encouragement, and others just need to know that someone cares. You may be the one who can help a mother, father, sister, brother, son, daughter, neighbor, or stranger who has struggled with the same problems that you had. Once you learn how to take care of yourself and act upon that knowledge, you can then pass your success on to others. You will then become a living testimony to the changes that are possible. What a tremendous opportunity!

The second greatest commandment is to love your neighbor as yourself. Caring about others is a Christian trait. Having the privilege to help others is a gift from heaven. Once you are able to get your health under control, it is an act of kindness and caring to help someone else who needs to get their health under control. You may be that person who has the privilege of helping someone before they develop a debilitating disease that could result in discomfort, massive medical expenses, or even premature death. Passing on to others those things that have been a blessing to you is the kind of giving that is Christlike.

Review these twelve principles. Think about how they relate to your own personal situation. Incorporate these principles into your daily life. Keep a journal, or at least a mental record, of the positive changes that have taken place since you made the changes that empowered you. It will be a helpful reminder to you as to why you made the changes in the first place. It will also be your testimony about the positive results that can be achieved after you decide to make changes in your life. Your changes can serve as a blueprint to help others that you come into contact with. Becoming healthy is really a pretty easy venture. The hard part is saying good-bye to the unhealthy habits that you have practiced for so long and saying hello to the new you. Now, let's get started!

Appendix

Body Mass Index

Body Mass Index Table

	Normal						Overweight					Obese										Extreme Obesity															
BMI	19	20	21	22	23	24	25	26	27	28	29	30	31	32	33	34	35	36	37	38	39	40	41	42	43	44	45	46	47	48	49	50	51	52	53	54
Height (inches)												Body Weight (pounds)																								
58	91	96	100	105	110	115	119	124	129	134	138	143	148	153	158	162	167	172	177	181	186	191	196	201	205	210	215	220	224	229	234	239	244	248	253	258
59	94	99	104	109	114	119	124	128	133	138	143	148	153	158	163	168	173	178	183	188	193	198	203	208	212	217	222	227	232	237	242	247	252	257	262	267
60	97	102	107	112	118	123	128	133	138	143	148	153	158	163	168	174	179	184	189	194	199	204	209	215	220	225	230	235	240	245	250	255	261	266	271	276
61	100	106	111	116	122	127	132	137	143	148	153	158	164	169	174	180	185	190	195	201	206	211	217	222	227	232	238	243	248	254	259	264	269	275	280	285
62	104	109	115	120	126	131	136	142	147	153	158	164	169	175	180	186	191	196	202	207	213	218	224	229	235	240	246	251	256	262	267	273	278	284	289	295
63	107	113	118	124	130	135	141	146	152	158	163	169	175	180	186	191	197	203	208	214	220	225	231	237	242	248	254	259	265	270	278	282	287	293	299	304
64	110	116	122	128	134	140	145	151	157	163	169	174	180	186	192	197	204	209	215	221	227	232	238	244	250	256	262	267	273	279	285	291	296	302	308	314
65	114	120	126	132	138	144	150	156	162	168	174	180	186	192	198	204	210	216	222	228	234	240	246	252	258	264	270	276	282	288	294	300	306	312	318	324
66	118	124	130	136	142	148	155	161	167	173	179	186	192	198	204	210	216	223	229	235	241	247	253	260	266	272	278	284	291	297	303	309	315	322	328	334
67	121	127	134	140	146	153	159	166	172	178	185	191	198	204	211	217	223	230	236	242	249	255	261	268	274	280	287	293	299	306	312	319	325	331	338	344
68	125	131	138	144	151	158	164	171	177	184	190	197	203	210	216	223	230	236	243	249	256	262	269	276	282	289	295	302	308	315	322	328	335	341	348	354
69	128	135	142	149	155	162	169	176	182	189	196	203	209	216	223	230	236	243	250	257	263	270	277	284	291	297	304	311	318	324	331	338	345	351	358	365
70	132	139	146	153	160	167	174	181	188	195	202	209	216	222	229	236	243	250	257	264	271	278	285	292	299	306	313	320	327	334	341	348	355	362	369	376
71	136	143	150	157	165	172	179	186	193	200	208	215	222	229	236	243	250	257	265	272	279	286	293	301	308	315	322	329	338	343	351	358	365	372	379	386
72	140	147	154	162	169	177	184	191	199	206	213	221	228	235	242	250	258	265	272	279	287	294	302	309	316	324	331	338	346	353	361	368	375	383	390	397
73	144	151	159	166	174	182	189	197	204	212	219	227	235	242	250	257	265	272	280	288	295	302	310	318	325	333	340	348	355	363	371	378	386	393	401	408
74	148	155	163	171	179	186	194	202	210	218	225	233	241	249	256	264	272	280	287	295	303	311	319	326	334	342	350	358	365	373	381	389	396	404	412	420
75	152	160	168	176	184	192	200	208	216	224	232	240	248	256	264	272	279	287	295	303	311	319	327	335	343	351	359	367	375	383	391	399	407	415	423	431
76	156	164	172	180	189	197	205	213	221	230	238	246	254	263	271	279	287	295	304	312	320	328	336	344	353	361	369	377	385	394	402	410	418	426	435	443

Body Mass Index Readings

Class	Body Mass Index
Severely underweight	Under 16.5
Underweight	16.5–18.4
Normal weight	18.5–24.9
Overweight	25.0–29.9
Obese	30.0–34.9
Clinically obese	35.0–39.9
Morbidly obese	40.0 and over[23]

Healthiest Foods to Consume

The majority of these foods contain at least several of the nutrients that our bodies need! They are among the richest sources of many of the essential nutrients needed for optimal health. Nutrient density is a measure of the amount of nutrients a food contains in comparison to the number of calories.

Vegetables	Fruits	Nuts and Seeds
Asparagus	Apples	Almonds
Avocados	Apricots	Cashews
Beets	Bananas	Flaxseeds
Bell Peppers	Blueberries	Olive oil
Broccoli	Cantaloupe	Peanuts
Brussels sprouts	Cranberries	Pumpkin seeds
Cabbage	Figs	Sesame seeds
Carrots	Grapefruit	Sunflower seeds
Cauliflower	Grapes	Walnuts
Celery	Kiwi fruit	
Collard greens	Lemon/limes	**Grains**
Cucumbers	Oranges	Barley
Eggplant	Papaya	Brown rice
Garlic	Pears	Buckwheat
Green beans	Pineapple	Corn
Green peas	Plums	Millet
Kale	Prunes	Oats
Leeks	Raisins	Quinoa
Mushrooms	Raspberries	Rye
Mustard greens	Watermelon	Spelt

		Whole wheat
Olives		Whole wheat
Onions		
Potatoes		
Romaine lettuce		
Spinach		
Squash, summer		
Squash, winter	**Beans and Legumes**	**Seafood**
Sweet potatoes	Black beans	Cod
Turnip greens	Garbanzo beans	Halibut
Yams	Kidney beans	Mahi Mahi
	Lentils	Orange Roughy
Spices and Herbs	Lima beans	Salmon
Basil	Miso	Perch
Black pepper	Navy beans	Trout
Cayenne pepper	Pinto beans	Tuna
Chili pepper, dried	Soybeans	
Cilantro	Tempeh	**Natural Sweeteners**
Cinnamon, ground	Tofu	Agave nectar
Cloves		Blackstrap molasses
Coriander seeds	**Low-Fat Dairy**	Cane juice
Cumin seeds	Almond milk	Honey
Dill	Cheese, low-fat	Liquid stevia
Dried peas	Eggs	Maple syrup
Ginger	Milk, 2 percent, cow	
Mustard Seed	Milk, goat	
Oregano	Milk, rice	
Parsley	Yogurt	

Peppermint		
Rosemary		
Sage	**Poultry and Lean Meat**	
Thyme	Beef, lean organic	
Turmeric	Calf's liver	
	Chicken	**Other**
	Lamb	Green tea
		Soy sauce (tamari)
		Water

To increase the number of nutrients that your body will receive and to maximize the value of these healthy foods, you should follow healthy preparation techniques. A healthy cooking method for vegetables is steaming. Steaming does not require the addition of butter, oils, or other fats. Steamed vegetables are healthy because they are softer and easier to digest then raw vegetables, and steaming allows vegetables to retain most of the vitamins, antioxidants, and other nutrients because the cooking time is short. Grilling is a healthy method for meat preparation. Grilling can provide exceptional taste with no added oils. Another healthy technique for cooking meat is roasting. By placing the meat on a rack in a pan, the meat will not be sitting in its own fat while roasting. Baking, broiling, and roasting are the healthiest ways to prepare poultry. Skinless poultry can be pan-broiled or stir-fried. You can use a nonstick pan or a nonstick spray coating. Poaching, steaming, baking, and broiling are the healthiest ways to prepare fish.

Sample Daily Eating Record

8:00 A.M.

Food	Calories	Protein	Carbs	Fats
Reduced-Fat Cottage Cheese	80	13	4	1.5
Blackberries	74	2	18	0.0
Whole-Grain Toast	60	2	12	0.5
Totals	**214**	**17**	**34**	**2.0**

11:00 A.M.

Food	Calories	Protein	Carbs	Fats
Chicken Breast (4 oz.)	140	33.5	0	3.5
Green Beans (double serving)	60	2.0	8	0.0
Blueberries (½ cup)	41	0.5	10	0.5
Totals	**241**	**36.0**	**18**	**4.0**

2:00 P.M.

Food	Calories	Protein	Carbs	Fats
Whole-Grain Bun	120	5	22	2
Barbeque Beef	140	22	0	6

Brussels Sprouts	60	4	14	0
Totals	**320**	**31**	**36**	**8**

5:30 P.M.

Food	Calories	Protein	Carbs	Fats
Baked Tilapia (5 oz.)	140	32	0	2
Baked Potato	143	3	34	0
Butter (½ serving)	37	0	0	4
Totals	**320**	**35**	**34**	**6**

8:30 P.M.

Food	Calories	Protein	Carbs	Fats
Strawberries	45	1	10	1
Pecans	200	3	4	20
Totals	**245**	**4**	**14**	**21**

Daily Totals

Calories	Protein	Carbs	Fats
1,340	**123**	**136**	**41**
Six servings of fruits or vegetables and six to ten glasses of water			

Note: You can find calorie, protein, carbohydrate, and fat content information on food labels or in the calorie counter books available in bookstores.

Recommended/Optimal Daily Intake

Vitamins

Key Nutrient	RDI	ODI
Vitamin A (Carotenes)	5,000 IU	5,000–25,000 IU
Vitamin B-1 (Thiamine)	1.5 mg	25–300 mg
Vitamin B-2 (Riboflavin)	1.7 mg	25–300 mg
Vitamin B-3 (Niacin)	20 mg	25–300mg
Vitamin B-5 (Pantothenic Acid)	10 mg	25–500 mg
Vitamin B-6 (Pyridoxine)	2 mg	25–300 mg
Vitamin B-9 (Folic Acid)	400 mcg	400–1,200 mcg
Vitamin B-12 (Cobalamin)	6 mcg	25–500 mcg
Vitamin B-15 (Pangamic Acid)	NA	25–100 mg
Vitamin C (Ascorbic Acid)	60 mg	500–5,000 mg
Vitamin D	400 IU	400–800 IU
Vitamin E	30 IU	400–1,200 IU
Vitamin K	80 mcg	80 mcg
Biotin	300 mcg	300 mcg
Choline	NA	50–500 mg
Inositol	NA	50–500 mg
PABA (Para-aminobenzoic Acid)	trace	30–100 mg

Minerals

KEY NUTRIENT	RDI	ODI
Boron	NA	3–6 mg
Calcium	1,000 mg	1,000–1,500 mg
Chromium	120 mcg	200–600 mcg
Copper	2 mg	05–25 mg
Iodine	150 mcg	150–300 mcg
Iron (Males)	10 mg	10–15 mg
Iron (Females)	18 mg	18–30 mg
Magnesium	400 mg	400–750 mg
Manganese	2 mg	15–30 mg
Molybdenum	75 mcg	75–500 mcg
Phosphorus	400 mg	400–1,000 mg
Potassium	99 mg	99–3,500 mg
Selenium	70 mcg	70–400 mcg
Zinc	15 mg	15–50 mg

Quantity Key

1. IU: International Units (a measurement for vitamins, dependent upon their potency)
2. mg: milligram; one-thousandth of a gram
3. mcg: microgram; one-millionth of a gram

Sample Workout Schedule

Monday: Upper body weight-resistance exercises
                (approximately forty-five minutes)

1. Do ten to fifteen minutes of light stretching before beginning the workout.
2. The lifting workout consists of four sets (three sets of the first exercise and one set of the second exercise) for each of the following body areas: chest, back, shoulders, biceps, and triceps.
3. The exercises listed below are only examples. You can exchange them or alternate them as long as the exercise exchanged is one that exercises the appropriate body area (i.e. change one back exercise for another back exercise, etc.).

   a. Bench press: 3 sets x 12 reps (1 min. rest between sets)
   b. Dumbbell fly: 1 set x 12 reps (2 min. rest after this set)
   c. Barbell or dumbbell bent-over rowing: 3 sets x 12 reps (1 min. rest between sets)
   d. Dumbbell reverse fly on a bench: 1 set x 12 reps (2 min, rest after this set)
   e. Dumbbell or barbell overhead press: 3 sets x 12 repetitions (1 min. rest between sets)
   f. Dumbbell lateral raise: 1 set x 12 reps (2 min. rest after this set)
   g. Dumbbell or barbell curl: 3 sets x 12 reps (1 min. rest between sets)
   h. Hammer curl: 1 set x 12 reps (2 min. rest after this set)
   i. Lying dumbbell extension: 3 sets x 12 reps (1 min. rest between sets)

    j.   Triceps kickback: 1 set x 12 reps (workout is completed after this set)

    k.   Do five to ten minutes of stretching after completing the workout.

Tuesday: Aerobic exercise (approximately twenty to sixty minutes in length but the shorter the workout, the greater the intensity should be)

1. Do ten to fifteen minutes of light stretching before beginning the workout.
2. Your choice of exercise may include swimming, jogging, running, using the elliptical machine, bicycling, participating in aerobic workout programs, jumping rope, or other aerobic choices.
3. Alternating exercises on aerobic workout days keeps the workouts from becoming monotonous.
4. Your heart rate should be between 60 to 85 percent of your maximum heart rate (220 minus your age) while doing the aerobic exercise.
5. If you cannot do aerobic exercise due to physical limitations, you should make this a walking workout. Do sixty minutes of walking per workout.
6. Do ten to fifteen minutes of stretching after completing the workout.

Wednesday: Lower body weight-resistance exercises (approximately forty-five minutes)

1. Do ten to fifteen minutes of light stretching before beginning the workout.
2. Squat: 3 sets x 12 reps. Without weight, holding dumbbells, or with a barbell and weights on your shoulders (1 min. rest between sets)
3. Lunge: 1 set x 12 reps. Holding dumbbells or without weight (2 min. rest after this set)

4. Dumbbell or barbell stiff-legged dead lift: 3 sets x 12 reps (1 min. rest between sets)
5. Leg curl: 1 set of 12 reps. Do this on a weight machine (2 min. rest after this set)
6. Toe raise holding dumbbells: 3 sets x 20 reps (1 min. rest after each set)
7. Toe raise: 1 set of 20 reps. Do this while seated with weight resting on your upper legs or standing while holding the weight and do toe raises with just one leg at a time (2 min. rest after this set)
8. Abdominal crunch: 3 sets of up to 50 reps per set. If this is not challenging enough, hold additional weight (weight plate or dumbbell) on your chest when completing repetitions (1 min. rest between sets)
9. Oblique crunch: 1 set of up to 50 reps
10. Do ten to fifteen minutes of stretching after completing the workout.

Thursday: Aerobic workout (twenty to sixty minutes). If physical limitations keep you from doing aerobic workouts, you should substitute the aerobics with sixty minutes of walking.

Friday: Repeat an upper body weight-resistance workout (like Monday). The repetitions remain the same, and exercises can remain the same or can be changed as long as they work the same body area.

Saturday: Aerobic workout (twenty to sixty minutes) using the same format as the Tuesday and Thursday workout.

Sunday: May either be a rest day or another aerobic workout like Tuesday, Thursday, or Saturday.

Workout Guidelines:

1. Work within your workout capabilities. It is important to challenge yourself but *only* within your fitness level. Work your way up to heavier weights and more intense aerobic workouts. In some cases it may be advisable to talk with your physician before beginning your program.

2. When lifting weights, attempt to work up to the heaviest weight that you can lift correctly for twelve repetitions. If you can do more than twelve, you are using too little weight. If you have to compromise good form to lift twelve repetitions of a weight or you are unable to complete twelve repetitions, you should be lifting a lighter weight until you can either lift that weight properly or complete the required number of repetitions. The goal is to get stronger *and* avoid injury. One technique is to lift your first set of twelve repetitions with a lighter weight and continue to add weight so that on your third set you are lifting the heaviest weight that you can lift properly for twelve repetitions.

3. Switch your aerobic workouts occasionally. Try different workouts for the sake of variety and different intensity levels.

4. On weight-resistance days alternate between upper body and lower body workouts. Example: if your last weight-resistance workout was upper body, then the next one will be lower body. Some weeks you will do two upper body workouts and one lower body workout, and the next week you will do two lower body workouts and one upper-body weight-resistance workout.

5. Record your workouts in a notebook so that you can refer back to it and see what weights you used (with what results) in previous workouts. This is helpful in planning future workouts.

Endnotes

Chapter 1: A Biblical Perspective Regarding Your Health

1. All Biblical quotes in this book are taken from the Old and New Testaments in the King James Version of the Holy Bible.

Chapter 2: What's the Big Deal?

1. *The Surgeon General's Report on Nutrition and Health.* United States Public Health Service, Office of the Surgeon General, 27 July 1988. Accessed Sept. 2010. <www.profiles.nlm.nih.gov.>.
2. *The Crisis Is Obesity.* United States Department of Human Services, 27 July 1988. Accessed Sept. 2010. <www.hhs.gov.>.
3. *Prevention of Childhood Overweight and Obesity.* United States Department of Human Services, Office of the Surgeon General, 11 Mar. 2008. Accessed Sept. 2010. <www.nhs.gov>.
4. *Obesity Health Care Costs US 147 Billion Dollars A Year, New Study.* Agency for Healthcare Research and Quality and the US Centers for Disease Control and Prevention (CDC), 28 July 2009. Accessed Sept. 2010. <www.medicalnewstoday.com>.
5. *Increases in Clinically Severe Obesity in the United States 1986–2000.* American Medical Association, 13 October 2003. Accessed Sept. 2010. < www.archinte.ama-assn. org>.
6. Ibid.
7. *Childhood Obesity: Most Experts Identified Physical Activity and the Use of Best Practices as a Key to Successful Programs.* United States Government Accountability

Office, 7 Oct. 2005. Accessed Sept. 2010. <www.gao.gov>.

8. Ibid.

9. *Discharged Servicemen Dispute Military Weight Rules.* Elizabeth Cohen and Elise Zeiger, 6 Sept. 2000. Accessed Sept. 2010. <www.cnn.com>.

10. *NIH in the 21st Century: The Director's Perspective.* Francis Collins, MD, PhD, Director National Human Genome Research Institute, U.S. Department of Health and Human Services. 15 June 2010. Accessed 2010. <www.hhs.gov>.

11. *Frequently Asked Questions About Calculating Obesity-Related Risk.* Centers for Disease Control and Prevention. 2005. Accessed September, 2010. <www.cdc.gov>.

12. *Innovations in Addressing Childhood Obesity.* Terry T-K Huang, PhD, MPH, Director Obesity Research Strategic Core. U.S. Department of Health and Human Services. 16 December 2009. Accessed Sept. 2010. <www.hhs.gov>.

13. *Health Topic: Obesity.* Medline Plus, 26 Aug. 2010. Accessed Sept. 2010. <www.medlineplus.gov>.

14. *Overweight and Obesity Trends Among Adults: Vital Signs: State-Specific Obesity Prevalence Among Adults–United States, 2009.* Centers for Disease Control and Prevention, 3 Aug. 2010. Accessed Sept. 2010. <www.cdc.gov>.

15. *Prevalence and Trends in Obesity Among U.S. Adults.* Katherine M. Flegal, PhD; Margaret D. Carroll, MSPH; Cynthia L. Ogden, PhD; Lester R. Curtin, PhD, *Journal of the American Medical Association*, 13 Jan. 2010. Accessed Sept. 2010. <www.jama.ama-assn.org>.

16. *Obesity in Children.* MedlinePlus, 24 Aug. 2010. Web Sept. 2010. <www.nlm.nih.gov/medlineplus/obesityinchildren>.

17. *Obesity and Nutrition Health Policy.* American Heart Association, 28 Aug. 2010. Accessed Sept. 2010. <www.heart.org>.
18. *Do Lifestyle Changes Improve Health?* World Health Organization, 9 Jan. 2009. Accessed August 2010.
19. *The World Health Report 2000–Health Systems: Improving Performance.* World Health Organization. 2000. Accessed Sept. 2010. <www.who.int/whr/2000>.
20. *National Health Expenditure Fact Sheet.* United States Department of Health and Human Services, Centers for Medicare and Medicaid Services, 29 June 2010. Accessed Sept. 2010. <www.cms.gov/NationalHealthExpendData>.
21. *Why We Eat….and Why We Keep Eating.* Dr. Jeffry Weiss, Sept. 2009. Accessed Sept. 2010. <www.insulitelabs.com>.
22. *Body Composition Tests.* American Heart Association, 29 Aug. 2010. Accessed Sept. 2010. <www.heart.org>.
23. *How Much Physical Activity for Everyone: Guidelines.* Centers for Disease Control and Prevention, May 2010. Accessed Sept. 2010. <www.cdc.gov>.
24. *Dietary Guidelines.* United States Department of Agriculture. 10 Sept. 2009. Accessed Sept. 2010. <www.mypyramid.gov>.

Chapter 3: A Picture of Health

1. *You: The Owner's Manual,* First ed. Michael F. Roizen, MD and Mehmet C. Oz, MD. New York: HarperCollins, 2008. Print.
2. Ibid.
3. *What is High Blood Pressure?* American Heart Association, 2 July 2009. Accessed Sept. 2009. <www.americanheart.org>.

4. *High Blood Pressure Dangers: Hypertension's Effects on Your Body.* Mayo Clinic Staff, 23 June 2009. Accessed Sept. 2009. <www.Mayoclinic.com>.
5. *Left Ventricular Hypertrophy.* Mayo Clinic Staff, 23 June 2009. Accessed Sept. 2009. <www.mayoclinic.com>.
6. *High Blood Pressure Dangers: Hypertension's Effects on Your Body.* Mayo Clinic Staff, 23 June 2009. Accessed Sept. 2009. <www.Mayoclinic.com>.
7. Ibid.
8. Ibid.
9. Ibid.
10. Ibid.
11. Ibid.
12. *High Blood Pressure Dangers: Hypertensions Effects on Your Body.* Mayo Clinic Staff, 8 July 2010. Accessed Sept. 2010. <www.Mayoclinic.com>.
13. *What is Glaucoma?* Prevent Disease, Sept. 2009. Accessed Sept. 2010. <www.preventdisease.com>.
14. *High Blood Pressure Dangers: Hypertensions Effects on Your Body.* Mayo Clinic Staff, 8 July 2010. Accessed Sept. 2010. <www.Mayoclinic.com>.
15. Ibid.
16. *Physical Activity.* American Heart Association, 23 Sept. 2010. Accessed Sept. 2010. <www.americanheart.org>.
17. *Resistance Training For High Blood Pressure!* Highbloodpressureinfo.org, 22 Sept. 2010. Accessed Sept. 2010. <www.highbloodpressureinfo.org>.
18. *Resting Heart Rate.* American Heart Association, 23 Sept. 2010. Accessed Sept. 2010. <www.americanheart.org>.
19. *Pulse.* MedlinePlus, 19 Aug. 2010. Accessed Sept. 2010. <www.nlm.nih.gov>.
20. *Benefits of Exercise.* Brian D. Johnston. The Merck Manuals Online Medical Library. Sept. 2007. Accessed Sept. 2010. <www.merck.com>.

21. *Resting Heart Rate.* American Heart Association, 23 Sept. 2010. Accessed Sept. 2010. <www.heart.org>.
22. *Target Heart Rates.* American Heart Association, 14 Sept. 2010. Accessed Sept. 2010. <www.americanheart. org>.
23. Ibid.
24. *Target Heart Rates.* American Heart Association, 23 Sept. 2010. Accessed Sept. 2010. <www.heart.org>.
25. *What Your Cholesterol Levels Mean.* American Heart Association, 2 July 2009. Accessed Sept. 2010. <www. americanheart.org>.
26. *High Cholesterol and Triglycerides.* Genesis Heart Institute, 2009. Accessed Sept. 2010. <www. genesishealth.com>.
27. *Prostate-Specific Antigen (PSA) Blood Test.* WebMD, Sept. 2009. Accessed Sept. 2010. <www.webmd.com>.
28. *Prostate-Specific Antigen (PSA) Test.* National Cancer Institute, 18 March 2009. Accessed Sept. 2010. <www. cancer.gov>.
29. *Extra Pounds Increase Arthritis Pain.* Carol and Richard Eustice, 24 May 2006. Accessed Sept. 2010. <www. arthritis.about.com>.
30. *How Regular Exercise Benefits Teens.* WebMD, 7 March 2010. Accessed Sept. 2010. <www.webmd.com>.
31. *Healthy Bones.* Dairy Council of California, 31 August 2010. Accessed Sept. 2010. <www.dairycouncilofca. org>.
32. *U.S. Spending on Health Care Slowed in 2008.* United States Department of Health and Human Services, 5 January 2010. Accessed Sept. 2010. <www. womenshealth.gov>.
33. Ibid.
34. *Recent Data on Health Insurance.* Centers for Disease Control and Prevention, 26 May 2010. Accessed Sept. 2010. <www.cdc.gov>.

35. *Assessing Your Weight and Health Risk.* U.S. Department of Health and Human Services, National Heart Lung and Blood Institute, 1 Sept. 2010. Accessed Sept. 2010. <www.nhlbi.nih.gov>.

36. *Why and How to Measure Your Body Fat Percentage.* Lynn VanDyke, 2009. Accessed Sept. 2010. <www.healthguidance.org>.

37. *What are the Guidelines for Percentage of Body Fat Loss?* Natalie Digate Muth, American Council on Exercise, 2 Dec. 2009. Accessed Sept. 2009. <www.acefitness.org>.

38. *Assessing Your Weight and Health Risk.* U.S. Department of Health and Human Services, National Heart Lung and Blood Institute, 1 Sept. 2010. Accessed Sept. 2010. <www.nhlbi.nih.gov>.

39. *Waist-Height Ratio May Show Heart Disease Risk.* Miranda Hitti. WebMD. 6 June 2005. Accessed Sept. 2010. <www.webmd.com>.

40. *The Truth About Fat.* WebMD, 23 Sept. 2010. Accessed Sept. 2010. <www.webmd.com>.

Chapter 4: So, I Want to Get Started ... Now What?

1. *List of Diets.* Wikimedia Foundation, Inc., 25 Aug. 2009. Accessed Sept. 2009. <www.en.wikipedia.org>.

2. *Diet Industry is Big Business.* Melissa McNamara, 1 Dec. 2006. Accessed Sept. 2010. <www.CBSnews.com>.

3. *Physical Activity and Your Heart.* National Institutes of Health, June 2006. Accessed Sept. 2010. <www.nhlbi.nih.gov>.

Chapter 5: Is All Food the Same?

1. *Steps to a Healthier You.* U.S. Department of Agriculture, 28 Aug. 2010. Accessed Sept. 2010. <www.MyPyramid.gov>.

2. *The Glycemic Index: The Key to Weight Loss and Optimal Fitness.* Travis Van Slooten, 2008. Accessed Sept. 2010. <www.menstotalfitness.com>.

3. *Personal Daily Calorie and Fat Limits.* American Heart Association, 9 Aug. 2010. Accessed Sept. 2010.

4. *Glycemic Index Chart.* Glycemic Edge. 26 Sept. 2010. Accessed Sept. 2010. <www.glycemicedge.com>.

5. *Dietary Guidelines for Americans 2005.* U.S. Department of Health and Human Services, 2005. Accessed Sept. 2010. <www.healthierus.gov/dietaryguidelines>.

6. Ibid.

7. *Trans Fats.* American Heart Association, Sept. 2010. Accessed Sept. 2010. <www.americanheart.com>.

8. *Nutrition for Everyone–Protein.* Centers for Disease Control and Prevention, 9 Nov. 2009. Accessed Sept. 2010. <www.cdc.gov>.

9. *Report of the Dietary Guidelines Advisory Committee on the Dietary Guidelines for Americans, 2010.* United States Department of Agriculture, 15 June 2010. Accessed Sept. 2010. <www.cnpp.usda.gov/Publications/DietaryGuidelines>.

10. *Water: How much Should You Drink Every Day?* Mayo Clinic Staff, 17 April 2010. Accessed Sept. 2010. <www.mayoclinic.com>.

11. *Signs and Symptoms of Dehydration.* Symptoms of Dehydration.com, Sept. 2010. Accessed Sept. 2010. <www.symptomsofdehydration.com>.

Chapter 6: You're Only as Healthy as Your Cells

1. *What is a Cell?* National Center for Biotechnology Information, 30 March 2004. Accessed Sept. 2010. <www.ncbi.nlm.nih.gov>.

2. Free Radical. *Merriam-Webster Dictionary*, 2010. Accessed Oct. 2010. <www.merriam-webster.com>.

3. *Oxidative Stress.* Thomas L. Clouse, MD, Aug. 2009. Accessed Sept. 2010. <www.walkingwithataxia.com>.
4. *Improving Health Through Antioxidants.* The Nutritional Foundation Program, Aug. 2010. Accessed Sept. 2010. <www.nutritionhouse.com>.
5. *USDA Database for the Oxygen Radical Absorbance Capacity (ORAC) of Selected Foods, Release 2.* U.S. Department of Agriculture, May 2010. Accessed Sept. 2010. <www.usda.gov>.
6. *Vitamin E.* Huntington's Outreach Project for Education, at Stanford, 3 May 2005. Accessed Sept. 2010. <www.stanford.edu>.
7. *Vitamin C.* National Institutes of Health, Office of Dietary Supplements, 12 Nov. 2009. Accessed Sept. 2010. <ods.od.nih.gov/factsheets/vitaminc.asp>.
8. *The Antioxidant Role of Glutathione and N-Acetyl-Cysteine Supplements and Exercise-Induced Oxidative Stress.* Chad Kerksick and Darryn Willoughby. *Journal of the International Society of Sports Nutrition*, 10 Nov. 2005. Accessed Sept. 2010. <www.ncbi.nlm.nih.gov>.

Chapter 7: Building Blocks For Life: Vitamins and Minerals

1. *Vitamin K.* Life Clinic International, Inc., Sept. 2010. Accessed Sept. 2010. <www.lifeclinic.com>.
2. National Institutes of Health, Office of Dietary Supplements, 24 August, 2007. Accessed Sept. 2010. <www.ods.od.nih.gov>.
3. *Fiber-O-Meter: Calculate the Fiber in Your Meals Each Day.* Kathleen M. Zelman, MPH, RD, LD, 22 Jan. 2010. Accessed Sept. 2010. <www.webmd.com>.
4. *The Seven Nutrients Americans are Most Deficient in and How to Get Them.* SixWise, 28 March 2007. Accessed Sept. 2010. <www.sixwise.com>.
5. Ibid.

6. Ibid.
7. Ibid.
8. Ibid.
9. Ibid.
10. *Vitamin and Mineral Guide*. African Holistic Healing Center, 2009. Accessed Sept. 2010. <u>www.drchism.com</u>.

Chapter 8: Do I Really Need to Exercise (The Answer is Yes!)

1. *Physical Activity*. American Heart Association, 30 Sept. 2010. Accessed Oct. 2010. <<u>www.americanheart.org</u>>.
2. *Physical Activity and Public Health in Older Adults: Recommendation*. American College of Sports Medicine, 2007. Accessed Sept. 2010. <<u>www.acsm.org</u>>.
3. *What Aerobic Exercise Does for Your Health*. Mayo Clinic Staff, 23 June 2009. Accessed Sept. 2010. <<u>www.mayoclinic.com</u>>.
4. *Maximum Heart Rate*. Sports Doctor, Inc., 2000. Accessed Sept. 2010. <<u>www.sportsdoctor.com</u>>.
5. *Fitness–Aerobic Fitness*. WebMd, 26 Aug. 2008. Accessed Sept. 2010. <<u>www.webmd.com</u>>.
6. *Walking for Fitness: How to Trim Your Waistline, Improve Your Health*. Mayo Clinic Staff, 23 June 2009. Accessed Sept. 2010. <<u>www.mayoclinic.com</u>>.
7. *Resistance Training–Beginners*. Better Health Channel, Nov. 2007. Accessed Sept. 2010. <<u>www.betterhealth.vic.gov</u>>.
8. *Stretching 101*. Laura Inverarity, DO, 7 Nov. 2007. Accessed Sept. 2010. <<u>www.physicaltherapy.about.com</u>>.

Chapter 9: Setting Goals

1. *Goal Setting–The Power of Writing Down Your Goal.* Raj In, 5 Nov. 2007. Accessed Sept. 2010. <<u>www.</u> <u>constantimprovements.com</u>>.

Chapter 10: What's Eating You?

1. *Percentage of Overweight, Obese Americans Swells.* Bill Hendrick. WebMD, 10 Feb. 2010. Accessed Sept. 2010. <<u>www.webmd.com</u>>.
2. <u>Love Hunger</u>, First ed. Dr. Frank Minirth, Dr. Paul Meier, Dr. Robert Hemfelt, Dr. Sharon Sneed, and Don Hawkins. New York: Ballantine Books, 1991. Print.
3. Ibid.
4. *Eating Triggers.* Weight Watchers, Jan. 2007.Accessed Sept. 2010. <<u>www.weightwatchers.com</u>>.
5. *Chocolate Cravings May Be Due to Magnesium Deficiency.* Kendall Scott. Portland Nutrition Examiner, 14 May 2009. Accessed Sept. 2010. <<u>www.examiner.com</u>>.

Appendix

1. *Body Mass Index Chart.* National Institutes of Health, Sept. 2010. Accessed Sept. 2010. < <u>www.nhlbi.nih.</u> <u>gov</u>>.